# LIFESTYLE RELATED DISEASES AMONG DOCTORS

## REETU SHARMA

# CONTENTS

## LIST OF TABLES

# ABBREVIATIONS

| | | |
|---|---|---|
| 'Doctor-patient' | : | Doctor who is suffering from illness |
| Physician of 'doctor-patient' | : | Doctor who is treating 'doctor-patient' |
| Doctor-patient | : | Doctor and Patient |
| WHO | : | World Health Organization |
| NCDs | : | Non-communicable Diseases |
| CVD | : | Cardio-vascular Diseases |
| COPD | : | Chronic Obstructive Pulmonary Disease |
| DM | : | Diabetes Mellitus |
| BP | : | Blood Pressure |
| HT | : | Hypertension |
| NPCDCS | : | National Programme for Cancer, Diabetes, Cardio-vascular and Stroke |
| NCRP | : | National Cancer Registry Programme |
| NTCP | : | National Tobacco Control Programme |
| RCCs | : | Regional Cancer Centres |
| NSSO | : | National Sample Survey Organization |
| GPs | : | General Practitioners |
| IMA | : | Indian Medical Association |
| PGIMER | : | Postgraduate Institution of Medical Education and Research |
| GDP | : | Gross Domestic Product |
| BMI | : | Body Mass Index |
| SEAR | : | South-east Asian Region |
| OPD | : | Out Door Patient |
| IPD | : | In Door Patient |
| NIDDK | : | National Institute of Diabetes, Digestive and Kidney Diseases |
| SPM | : | Social and Preventive Medicine |
| ENT | : | Ear, Nose and Trachea |
| GOI | : | Government of India |

# CHAPTER I

## INTRODUCTION

Culture plays an important in shaping the lifestyle of the people in a society. It provides the choices to the people that shape the daily habits of the people. Lifestyle of people can be healthy or unhealthy depending upon the choices they make in their day to day life. Healthy lifestyle is conducive to physical and mental wellbeing of a person while unhealthy lifestyle leads to lifestyle related diseases. Thus, lifestyle related diseases once seen as pathological in origin are now considered to be influenced by the lifestyle of the people.

Developed and developing societies all over world are being affected by lifestyle related diseases (World Health Organization [WHO], 2011). The most common lifestyle related diseases are diabetes, cancer, cardio-vascular and respiratory diseases. The incidence as well as the mortality rate due to lifestyle related diseases is rising in nearly all the countries. The lifestyle of the people is considered to be important in finding out the presence of various risk factors causing the lifestyle related diseases. WHO considers unhealthy diet, lesser physical activity, use of tobacco products and excessive intake of alcohol as the most important risk factors. These risk factors are generally modifiable and also known as behavior risks factors because these factors are reflected in the lifestyle and daily habits of the people. In addition, obesity, hypertension and stress are considered other factors increasing the risk of lifestyle related diseases.

Moreover, unhealthy lifestyle such as unhealthy diet, excessive use of alcohol, lack of physical activity, use of tobacco, stress etc. decreases the body immunity to fight the diseases and thus, possibility of development of lifestyle related diseases increases. Studies also show that healthy lifestyle plays an important role in keeping oneself healthy and in contrast to this, unhealthy lifestyle results in to onset of a number of lifestyle related diseases.

All the sections of society are vulnerable to these diseases. Medical professionals, particularly the doctors are expected to be extra conscious with regard to their health. It is often assumed that lifestyle of a doctor will be healthy as compared to an ordinary person. They are considered to be quite knowledgeable about the healthy and balanced diet and negative impact of physical inactivity, excessive use of alcohol, cigarette smoking, stress etc. on the health. But the risk factors responsible for these diseases seem to be equally present among doctors also.

The present research tries to fill the gap in the existing literature relating to sociological causes and consequences of lifestyle related diseases among the doctors in Punjab. We tried to look into the lifestyle of the doctors and its relation to the presence of diverse risk factors and habits responsible for the occurrence of lifestyle related diseases. The study is also important as social consequences of lifestyle related diseases have not been studied much.

It is important to understand concept of Health, Lifestyle, and Lifestyle related diseases in order to make an attempt to study the lifestyle related diseases among doctors.

**HEALTH**

According to Dubos, "health can be defined as the ability to function" (as cited in Cockerham, 1986, p.3). Good health is the essence of a balanced relationship of mind and body with regard to social and physical environment. In modern times, medical field is focused on the health problems of a person as a whole rather than in parts.

Cockerham (1986) observes that in the present time, the main cause of health-related problems can be traced in to 'problems in living' related to the socio-cultural and psychological environment in addition to the biological, physiological and pathological factors (Cockerham, 1986).

What are the reasons behind the health problems of an individual, what is the experience as being sick, and how the coping mechanism takes place? All of these questions cannot be answered without considering the prevailing socio-cultural environment present in the society and expectations of behavior according to that particular societal environment. There are number of factors that act as social determinants of health and are useful in avoidance of disease. Overall wellbeing of a person depends upon the interplay of numerous factors existing equally in biological makeups of the person as well as in the society.

The model by Dahlgren and Whitehead (1991) explains interaction between different causal factors right from individual and community levels to the level of health policies that result in health inequalities. This model illustrates the following factors in the form of four layers which are as follows:

a) At the centre: Age, gender and genetic factors.

b) First layer: Person's lifestyle or behavior factors.

c) Second layer: Social and community networks.

d) Third layer: Living and working atmosphere e.g. accommodation, work surroundings, education, healthcare services etc.

e) Fourth layer: Social, cultural, economic and environmental factors present in the society.

A numbers of studies carried out on the relationship between social conditions and emergence of a disease have also come up with the same observations as given by Dahlgren and Whitehead Model. World Health Organization also recognized the importance of social factors present in the society for the wellbeing of people and came forward with the formation of 'Commission on Social Determinants of Health' in the year 2008 to address the issue of social inequities.

Since the study is focused on the lifestyle related diseases, it is essential to comprehend the sociological conceptualization of Lifestyle.

**LIFESTYLE**

'Lifestyle' generally involves the attitudes, opinions, interests, and behaviors of an individual, a group and a culture. The 'lifestyle' shows variations according to gender, age, education, income, place of living (rural or urban), caste, race, religion, and ethnicity. The people belonging to different age groups, gender, income and education groups, caste, religion, rural and urban settings differ in their attitudes, thinking, behaviors, areas of interests, opinions, eating habits, dressing style, living style etc. In social interaction, lifestyle becomes a medium by which a person projects one's place in 'status hierarchy'. In nutshell, we can say the people belonging to different groups have different 'way of living'.

A number of thinkers have different perceptions about the concept of 'lifestyle'.

Veblen (1899) observes that people follow specific 'schemes of life' i.e. lifestyle on the basis of their desire to show compliance to a stratum which is considered to be superior to them and to make a distance from the strata that is believed to be inferior to them.

Weber (1921) states that lifestyle is the 'concrete' and 'visible' manifestation of status groups. Lifestyle is reflected by the status or prestige of an individual and a group. So, the lifestyle results in to social differentiation even within the same social class.

Bourdieu (1984) analyses that lifestyle consists of social practices ingrained in social structure and adherence of people choices to these social practices. So, Bourdieu talks about the interaction between the 'Structure' and 'Agency'.

Hence, from the above discussion, it can be concluded that lifestyle is sum total of all the activities, functions, behaviours we do in our day to day life such as activities related to our work, our leisure activities, eating habits, interaction activities with other people like family members, colleagues, friends, neighbours, peer group etc.

Further, lifestyle and health of the individual are strongly linked to each other. The health of a person depends upon the lifestyle that he or she follows. Lifestyle may be healthy or unhealthy. A healthy lifestyle results in to satisfactory, healthy and happy life while an unhealthy lifestyle leads to emergence of health related problems. Scholars have valued the role of healthy lifestyle for the overall wellbeing of people. Healthy lifestyle leads to 'enhance health and life expectancy' (Cockerham, 1998). In addition, McAmmond (2000) revealed that probability of emergence of chronic diseases, disability and premature death is directly linked to poor nutrition.

**LIFESTYLE RELATED DISEASES**

Lifestyle related diseases are caused due to an inappropriate and imbalance relationship of people with their environment. They are mainly concerned with the daily habits of people. These diseases are of long duration, slow progression, not completely treatable and non-communicable in nature. The other synonyms used for these diseases are 'chronic diseases', 'non-communicable diseases', 'diseases of affluence', 'diseases of civilization', 'diseases of longevity' etc.

WHO (2005a) stated that lifestyle related diseases are not solely the result of genetic factors and individual's behavior but the environmental factors such as physical, socio-cultural and economic factors also have marked effect for the emergence of these diseases.

WHO enlisted the following factors for the causation of these diseases:

- Socio-cultural, economic, political and environmental determinants.

- Risk factors: A 'risk factor' is the factor that increases the risk of developing a disease on exposure to that particular factor.

According to WHO (2005), risk factors are important indicator in predicting the likelihood of occurrence of a disease. These are divided in to following parts:

a) Modifiable or Behaviour risk factors such as physical inactivity, unhealthy diet, smoking, harmful consumption of alcohol.

b) Non-modifiable risk factors like gender, age, genetic factors, ethnicity.

c) Intermediate risk factors including high blood pressure level, high sugar level, obesity, abnormal lipid profile.

In addition to above risk factors, there are some other risk factors like environmental risk factors (environmental pollutants), cultural factors (lifestyle, beliefs, practices) and socio-economic risk factors (income, education, social and community networks) that are important in the development of diseases.

## MAJOR LIFESTYLE RELATED DISEASES

According to WHO (1999), there are four major lifestyle related diseases. These are heart diseases, respiratory diseases, diabetes and cancer. In addition to these four major lifestyle diseases, arthritis, spondylitis, hypertension, osteoporosis, stroke etc. are also associated with the faulty lifestyle among individuals.

### Cardiovascular Disease (CVD)

CVD involves the diseases related to heart and blood vessels. WHO (2011a) found that one third of all the deaths are owing to heart diseases globally and in case of deaths due to NCDs (non-communicable diseases) share of heart diseases is half.

Xavier et al. (2008) claimed that the Indian people suffer from heart diseases at much earlier age as compared to the people of developed nations. The article also projected sixty percent of India's share in the global burden of heart diseases in the coming two years.

**Diabetes Mellitus**

Diabetes is caused when insulin is not produced and secreted properly by pancreas. Insulin is essential to control the blood sugar level in the body. Inadequate secretion of insulin results in to high sugar level in the body. Diabetes increases the chances of emergence of other diseases such as kidney diseases, heart diseases, eye diseases, blindness etc.

The presence of diabetes is found to be directly linked to the social and economic status of the countries. The incidence of diabetes is the lowest in low income countries i.e. eight percent and the highest for upper middle-income countries i.e. ten percent (WHO, 2011a). India has been projected as 'Diabetes Capital' and the figure of diabetic patients will touch seventy million by 2025.

**Cancer**

Cancer is the rapid and abnormal division of body cells. Cancer stands second after heart diseases globally as far as mortality is concerned. It is an estimation that the number of people suffering from cancer will rise to 21.4 million in 2030 (WHO, 2011a). The share of low and middle-income countries will be two-third of these patients.

Women mainly suffer from breast, uterus, ovaries and cervix cancers while in men the cancers of lungs, oesophagus and oral cavity are mostly prevalent. Tobacco consumption both smoking and smokeless and excessive intake of alcohol are two leading behaviour factors that increase the risk of cancer.

**Chronic Obstructive Pulmonary Disease (COPD)**

The major behavior risk factor responsible for COPD is tobacco use. The estimated number for COPD patients was 22 million by 2016 as compared to 13 million in 1996 in India (National Commission on Macroeconomics and Health, 1996-2016).

In addition to above major chronic diseases, there are also some chronic conditions which are associated with the lifestyle of people like chronic backache, spondylitis, stress, insomnia, hypertension, osteoporosis etc.

**PREVALENCE OF LIFESTYLE RELATED DISEASES IN INDIA**

Nowadays lifestyle related diseases are showing a rising trend at the international, national and regional level which is reflected in the reports published from time to time. Some of the reports mentioning the burden and mortality due to lifestyle related diseases in India are given as follows:

**a) Non-Communicable Diseases and their Risk Factors in India**

There is an increase in mortality (deaths) and morbidity (illness) due to non-communicable diseases in India. This is confirmed by the excerpts from Global Status Report on burden of non-communicable diseases and their risk factors in India (WHO, 2014). Some of the facts mentioned in this report points towards the alarming situation prevailing in India are:

- Overall mortality due to non-communicable diseases (NCDs) in India is sixty percent (5.87 million). The mortality due to NCDs in India is more than two-third of mortality in the South-East Asian Region (SEAR).

- The highest mortality rate is due to cardiovascular diseases (45%) followed by chronic respiratory disease (22 %), cancers (12 %) and diabetes (3%).

- The worst hit is the productive population of the country that lies in the age group of 30-70 years that results into economic burden on the country.

- Tobacco consumption is the single largest risk factor responsible for all the major non-communicable diseases.

- In 2010, the per capita (age 15 and above) utilization of pure alcohol in India (4.3 litres per year) was much higher than the average consumption in South East Asian Region (3.2 litres per year).

- In India, raised blood glucose level is found in every tenth person and raised blood pressure level is found in every fourth person aged 18 years or above.

**b) Comparison of Statistics related to Causes of Mortality in India in 2005 and 2030**

The Table 1.1 given below shows the statistics related to causes of mortality in India in 2005 and projections of these causes of mortality in 2030. The Table shows the accerlation of mortality rate due to various non-communicable diseases over a period of twenty-five years. For instance, an increase in mortality rate due to cardio-vascular diseases is expected to be approximately seven percent whereas for cancer the rise is of nearly four percent and there is three percent increase in mortality rate due to other chronic conditions in 2030. Importantly, mortality rate due to communicable diseases shows a downward trend from 2005 to 2030.

**Table 1.1 Major Causes of Death in India (in Percentage) in 2005 and 2030**

| Year | Cardiovascular Diseases | Cancer | Other Chronic Conditions | Communicable Diseases | Injuries |
|------|-------------------------|--------|--------------------------|-----------------------|----------|
| 2005 | 29.00% | 8.00% | 16.00% | 36.20% | 10.80% |
| 2030 | 35.90% | 11.90% | 19.10% | 21.00% | 12.10% |

Source: WHO, 2011a.

**INITIATIVES TAKEN BY GOVERNMENT OF INDIA**

From the above given facts it becomes clear that lifestyle related diseases and their risk factors are increasing day by day in India. Ministry of Health and Family welfare, Government of India took many initiatives by starting a number of different programs to address this issue. The initiatives taken by Government of India are as follows:

**a) 'National Programme for Prevention and Control of Cancer, Diabetes, Cardio-vascular Diseases and Stroke' (NPCDCS)**

This programme was initiated in 2007 as a pilot project in the states of Assam, Andhra Pardesh, Gujarat, Kerala, Karnatka, Madhya Pardesh, Punjab, Rajasthan, Sikkim, and Tamil Nadu. The main objectives of this programme are to prevent and to early detect the above said non-communicable diseases. This programme focuses to generate awareness for the change in daily habits of people and to upgrade the healthcare system to make them efficient to tackle NCDs.

**b) 'National Cancer Control Programme'**

This programme was initiated in 1975. The recommendations made under this program are to recognize the new 'Regional Cancer Centres' (RCCs), to provide the financial aid to government institutions for developing the cancer treatment centre and 'District Cancer Control Programmers' at district levels.

**c) 'National Cancer Registry Programme' (NCRP)**

This programme was started in 1982. The main objective of this programme is to monitor the incidence of cancer and emerging trends in cancer prevalence in India.

**d) 'National Trauma Control Programme'**

To address the problem of increasing number of injuries due to road accidents, Ministry of Health and Family Welfare came up with this programme. The main components of this programme are pre-hospital trauma care, hospital care, rehabilitation of patient etc.

**e) 'National Programme for Control of Blindness'**

This programme was started in 1976. Main targets of this programme is to bring the blindness rate to 0.3 % by 2020, to clear the backlog of eye patients, to generate awareness about the healthy eye care practices, to establish well equipped healthcare system, to encourage the participation of non-government organizations and eye specialist in private practice to address this issue.

**f) 'The National Tobacco Control Programme'** (NTCP)

This programme was started in 2007-2008. The main parts constituting this NTCP programme are: i) to generate awareness among people about the damaging effects of tobacco consumption ii) to monitor effective implementation of law related to tobacco control at district level iii) to upgrade the present laboratories for testing tobacco products and iv) to monitor and evaluate 'Tobacco Control Programme' regularly.

**LIFESTYLE RELATED DISEASES IN PUNJAB**

The prevalence of morbidity (illness) in Punjab in 2004 was 127 per 1000 people as against the figure of 91 per thousand people at all India level (NSSO, 2006). Thus, the morbidity of Punjab was found to be more than the national average. According to this data, Punjab was found to be the second largest morbidity state in India, next only to Kerala.

A survey of 5,127 people within an age group of 18-69 years was undertaken in 2014-2015 in Punjab by PGI (Chandigarh) along with four medical colleges of state (Amritsar medical college, Patiala medical college, Faridkot medical college, Dayanand medical college) for measuring the risk factors for non-communicable diseases (PGIMER, 2014). It is known as STEPS Survey because it was performed in three steps to measure risk factors related to lifestyle related diseases. These three steps were a) to measure the behavior risk factors like unhealthy diet, tobacco consumption etc. b) physical measures like height, body weight etc. c) biochemical measures like blood glucose level, cholesterol level, lipid profile etc.

This survey indicated that there is high prevalence of risk factors which can result in to lifestyle related diseases among adults in Punjab. It was found that all the four recognized risk factors including tobacco consumption, excessive intake of alcohol, unhealthy diet and low physical activity are present in high percentage among the people of Punjab.  The most alarming fact that reflects the grim situation of NCDs in Punjab is that only one percent of population under study was free from any above said risk factors.

The above explained facts point towards the critical situation related to lifestyle related or non-communicable diseases in India and especially in Punjab. Now in such a scenario, the health of an individual is the main concern for over all development of a nation or a state. And health of the doctors is the major concern because if the people related to the medical profession will be healthy, they will provide the quality care to their patients. So to act on the health front and to fight against the diseases, health of the doctors is very important to have a healthy society.

**LIFESTYLE AND HEALTH AMONG DOCTORS**

It is expected that doctors are healthier as compared to the common people (Schlicht, Gordon, Ball & Christie, 1990). But Kay, Michell & Del (2004) established that the rates of chronic illness as well as preventive health needs are same like the general community among doctors.

Lifestyle habits of doctors reflect that doctors ignore their health needs like common man. Doctors do not follow the healthy dietary pattern and regular exercise schedule. Besides unhealthy diet and physical inactivity, the other factors (excessive intake of alcohol and smoking) responsible for lifestyle related diseases are also present in doctors. Lewy (1986) and Juntunen et al. (1988) in their studies mentioned the habits of excessive intake of alcohol among doctors whereas prevalence of smoking habits among doctors in Malaysian hospital was observed by Yaccob and Abdulha (1993).

The unhealthy lifestyle may be due to the work culture among doctors where they have to fulfill their professional commitments in preference to their personal obligations. This unhealthy lifestyle at the end has marked effect on their mental and physical health. The studies show that doctors are also a biological and social being and they are also susceptible to unhealthy lifestyle like common man and ultimately fall prey to diseases.

Thus, doctors who are considered as the gate keeper to the diseases are not immune to the diseases and their social, economic and psychological impacts like common man. They too have a feeling of uneasiness, segregation and being cut off from normal life during the phase of illness. Chronic illness leads to loneliness and isolation among doctors (Wessely & Gerada, 2013) and as a result of this, doctors have to  keep themselves away from practice and thus, a feeling of isolation from their peer group comes to them (Tomalinson, 2014). Also, denial attitude towards illness inhibits doctors in seeking care for themselves (McKall, 2001).

However, the phase of being sick sometimes plays a positive role in the lives of doctors. This phase transforms the doctors in to better professionals. Now they can understand very well the feeling and suffering of a person while passing through that critical phase of illness on the one hand and expectations lying in the doctor-patient relationship from patient's perspective on the other hand (Benziman, Kannai & Ahmad, 2012;  Wessely & Gerada , 2013). But this is also observed that if the health of the doctor is impaired it is not good for the health and safety of the patient because he will not be able to provide good care to patients (Firth-Cozens, 2001)

Hence, high rate of mortality and morbidity due to lifestyle related diseases and healthcare issue of doctors have emerged as an important area of concern these days. Normally it is understood that doctors are expert in following healthy lifestyle by taking healthy and balanced diet, doing regular exercise, avoiding bad habits that can have ill effect on their health. But above given observations presented a different picture about the health, lifestyle and attitude of doctors towards illness.

So, the irregularities related to lifestyle lead to physical and psychological manifestation of a large number of health related problems. This unhealthy lifestyle in the form of imbalanced diet, physical inactivity, alcohol and tobacco consumption, anxiety, lack of sleep, stress etc. lead to lifestyle related diseases like heart problems, breathing troubles, cancer and diabetes mellitus.

**STATEMENT OF PROBLEM**

The reasons for disease may be genetic as well as social. The efforts to deal with diseases are required at both levels. Further, research studies indicate that besides the biological reasons, the unhealthy lifestyle of individuals is also a major cause for some non-communicable diseases such as heart ailments, respiratory diseases, diabetes and cancer. These diseases are thus known as lifestyle related diseases. In addition to the four major lifestyle diseases, the arthritis, spondylitis, hypertension, osteoporosis, stroke etc. are also linked to the faulty lifestyle among individuals. The present study thus tries to focus on understanding the socio-economic and cultural causes and consequences of lifestyle related diseases.

The mortality rate for lifestyle related diseases, also termed as non-communicable diseases, is high in all parts of the world. The projections show that South Asian region of which India is a part will have the highest rise in mortality rate of 21 % i.e. 51% to 72% from 2008-2030 (Nikolic, Stanciole & Zaydman, 2011). World Health Organization (2002) found that sixty percent of the deaths all over world in 2001 were from four diseases, i.e. cancer, diabetes, heart and respiratory diseases. On the other hand, only forty percent of the deaths were caused by infectious or communicable diseases like AIDS, tuberculosis and malaria etc. The report claims that enough attention has not been given to the prevention and treatment of these diseases. Such an investment in dealing with chronic diseases is a vital necessity according to this report.

The magnitude of the problem can also be understood in terms of the economic loss due to these diseases. According to Abegunde & Stanciole (2006), there is an estimation of loss of national income equivalent to US $23 billion as a result of mortality due to three chronic conditions (diabetes, heart diseases and stroke) in India over a span of ten years i.e. from 2005-2015. India stands second on income loss as a percentage of GDP (1.27% of GDP) in 2015 among nine countries second to Russia which was expected to suffer a loss of 5.34% of GDP due to NCDs in 2015 (Abegunde & Stanciole, 2006). This economic loss is attributed to both direct cost (medical expenses for medicines and laboratory tests) and indirect cost (disability adjusted life years, loss of labour, cost incurring in providing care to the sick member etc.) while managing these diseases.

The main reason behind the rise in mortality rate and high economic loss due to lifestyle related diseases is the defective lifestyle. The process of globalization, industrialization and urbanization bring with it a drastic change in lifestyle of people. This change in lifestyle of people is seen in every part of life. For instance, a change is visible in daily eating habits, dressing style, way of living, work culture, social and community ties as well as in the norms, values and attitudes of the people. Thus, these processes have affected both material and non-material culture of Indian society.

As stated earlier, risk of having lifestyle related diseases increases due to practice of unhealthy lifestyle. This unhealthy lifestyle has penetrated in food habits of people resulting into a transition in eating habits of people. Eating habits of people shifted to a culture of processed food in the form of fast and junk food which have high level of sugar, salt, fat and calories. This high level of calories and fat result in to increase in body weight. Moreover, high level of sugar and salt present in processed food result in to increase in sugar and blood pressure level respectively. Thus, increase in body weight, high blood sugar and blood pressure level lead to lifestyle related diseases like diabetes, heart diseases, cancer etc.

In addition to the unhealthy food habits, the physical inactivity due to excessive mechanization resulted in to causation of a number of health related problems. Machines have dominated every sphere of personal as well as professional life equally in rural and urban areas. Machines have replaced the man power. Previously the works which were done manually are now done with machines. The use of machines for various pursuits has reduced the physical labour that resulted in to decrease in physical activity and therefore, a sedentary lifestyle among people.

Even leisure activities are not being spared from the bad effects of technology. Indoor leisure activities like watching television, playing computer games and excessive use of internet have replaced the outdoor leisure activities. This further resulted in to escalation of sedentary lifestyle and physical inactivity. Moreover, overindulgence for computer and mobile phones interfere with the healthy sleep pattern of an individual. Required amount of seven to eight hours of sleep is essential for the physical as well as mental health of people.

Further, indoor leisure activities have also affected the mental and emotional health of people by reducing the social interaction among people. Man is social animal and being gregarious is the basic nature of the human-beings. In present time, most of the physical and mental problems are the result of lack of interaction between the individuals.

Also, the process of globalization brought with it a sea change in the work culture of people. In today's life the materialistic pursuits to earn more and more money dominate the person that lead to increase in physical and psychological stress. Booming of multi-national companies brought with it a culture of long working hours at odd periods of time and target oriented approach. This has a striking effect on physical and mental wellbeing of people.

Besides propagating the culture of unhealthy food habits, sedentary and materialistic lifestyle, the process of urbanization and industrialization brought with it overcrowding of the urban spaces and polluted environment due to heavy vehicular traffic. The pollutants emitted by these industries and motor vehicles are the big cause of breathing, lung, heart problems and cancer.

The above given lifestyle changes of people in the form of physical inactivity, unhealthy food, stress etc. affected each and every strata of society. Consequently, there is an increase in prevalence of lifestyle related health problems and high rate of mortality and morbidity due to these troubles.

From the above discussion, it appears that heart diseases, various types of cancers, psychological and nervous disorders, thus, the big reasons of morbidity (illness) and mortality (deaths) are not only due to the problem of endogenous (internal) biological processes taking place in the body but also of exogenous (external) agents present in society. Further, WHO (2005a) states that eighty percent of cardiovascular diseases, stroke and diabetes and more than forty percent of cancers are preventable by observing a healthy lifestyle. So there is an important relationship between social-cultural and economic environment (housing, diet, urban space and occupation) and development of disease.

The present research is focused on the lifestyle related diseases among doctors in Punjab. The statistics show that lifestyle related diseases are increasing at an alarming rate at national and international level. These diseases have direct relationship with behavior risk factors such as excessive intake of alcohol, physical inactivity, unhealthy diet and tobacco use. Thus the people with these behavior risk factors are at higher risk of suffering from these diseases.

Lifestyle related diseases are penetrating every section and strata of society. Doctors constitute an important section of the society and this section of society is considered to be the most conscious about their lifestyle and they are assumed to follow a healthy lifestyle. But the facts show that risk factors for lifestyle related diseases are present in doctors in the same proportion as in an ordinary man. So, doctors who are considered as 'custodian of health' of the society are also at risk of development of lifestyle related diseases.

Now in such a scenario, the health of doctors is important for the health of society, if doctors are not healthy and they are not observing the preventive measures to avoid the lifestyle related diseases, then it will become difficult for them to provide good and quality healthcare to the patients. So, present study is an effort to know about the health status of doctors with reference to lifestyle related diseases, reasons behind following an unhealthy lifestyle, experiences of doctors when they become patients and coping mechanism adopted by them in case of suffering from lifestyle related diseases.

The study is carried in Punjab as the Punjabis are famous for their fondness for food and their eating habits. Further, morbidity in Punjab is high as compared to average morbidity at all India level. Also, the emerging and changing urban culture of busy and stressful life with inadequate physical activity and rest necessitates such a study particularly amongst the doctors who are considered to be most aware and informed about the causes and consequences of the lifestyle related diseases in general.

**THEORETICAL FRAMEWORK**

Several theories and models have been used to explain the origin and impact of diseases. The perspectives in sociology have tried to focus on the individual as well as systematic dimensions of diseases and health of individuals in society. Some of the models and perspectives are discussed underneath.

Traditionally there have been two models to understand and explain the origin and development of diseases. The two models were 'Bio-medical' and 'Social model'. Apart from these two models, several perspectives can be applied to understand the phenomenon. They are functional, interactionism, social-psychological, post-modern perspectives and health lifestyle theory.

As sociologists we are more interested in the social model that focuses on social determinants of health and diseases. However, Germov (2009) explained that the transition from 'Biomedical Model' to 'Social Model' took years. A brief explanation of the two models by Germov, their limitations and importance is given below:

**The Biomedical Model**

The biomedical model is based upon the idea of 'germ theory of disease' which focuses on the role of germs in causing a disease. The theory was propounded by Louis Pasteur in 1978. Later, Robert Koch developed a new term 'specific aetiology' that was founded on the thought that every disease is caused by a specific kind of bacteria. The spread of these disease causing bacteria may take place through food, air, water etc. and thus, communicable in nature.

The biomedical model brought with it a significant advancement in diagnosing and treating the communicable diseases which were the major cause for mortality at that time. But the biological model has a number of shortcomings such as treating the body like a machine and is mainly concerned with the repair of only diseased parts, considers human biology as the single cause for development of illness and ignoring social and psychological factors for the causation of disease (Dubos, 1959).

This single cause or mono-causal model of disease was a dominant model of early twentieth century. According to Najman (1980) in twentieth century medical field was mainly focused on the diagnosis and curing of specific diseases in individuals. There was no reference to social causes of origin of disease. Thus, medical field in western societies was predominantly interested in biological reasons rather than social reasons for the origin of disease.

**The Social Model**

Bio-medical model that depends upon medical treatment in improving health of people was criticized by McKeown (1979). He stressed that rather than treating a disease with medicine, preventive measures should be put by altering the circumstances that lead to the onset of diseases. This led to the development of the 'Social model' of health. Social model also values the importance of biological and psychological factors and role of medicine in treating the diseases in consonance with the social factors.

Germov (2009) also came to the conclusion that although individual (agency)-based and structure-based approaches have their basis in the biomedical and the social model of health respectively, but despite of their dissimilar genesis, they are interconnected and cannot be separated.

Thus bio-model and social model exist side by side with their different areas of interests regardless of having a situation of conflict between the 'structure and agency' in causation of a disease. The biomedical model focuses on treating the disease biologically focusing only on working of the human body while social model explores the inequalities in health based on sex, ethnicity, income, caste, occupational status etc. in the society.

The World Health Organization (WHO, 1946) recognized the importance of social as well as physical and mental well-being and defined health as "a state of complete physical, mental and social well-being and not merely the absence of disease or infirmity". Thus, WHO emphasized the importance of overall 'well-being' of people rather than merely absence of an   illness.

Apart from the above models, several perspectives can be used to explain the origin and impact of lifestyle related diseases

**Structural-Functionalist Perspective**

The main proponent of this tradition is Parsons (1951). The key emphasis of this perspective is the function of various items towards maintaining social order and stability. This can result from the shared values. According to Parsons, health is functional for the society and sickness is deviance i.e. dysfunctional for the society. The main focus of this approach is to explain the chronic illness from functional disabilities point of view.

Parson's sick role concept was mainly used to focus upon the social aspects related to living with the acute diseases. Sick role is the temporary condition where the person changes his or her normal lifestyle and adopts a changed lifestyle.  Such a person is supposed to withdraw from normal activities, take sufficient rest and adhere to the advice of a physician.  This leads to recovery from an illness and normalization of life.

In addition to the Parson's concept that health is functional for the society, Durkheim stressed that social and community ties are functional for the health of an individual. Durkheim (1966) provided the argument that "social and community networks and social stress are very important in lowering and increasing the probability of illness."

**Interactionist Perspective**

This is based on the contributions made by Mead (1934) and Blumer (1969). This perspective deals with the micro-level interaction between the individuals. Here the focus shifts from 'Structure' to 'Agency'. The experience and perception of the actor is given importance in this perspective.

Human beings have the ability to think and define a situation. As a result of this continuous process of thinking and interpretation, the people interact. Thus, social life comes in to being as a result of interaction among the individuals who chose their own behavior and finally act accordingly.

Goffman (1959) described the experience of being sick from patient's perspective. According to him, illness of long duration affects thought process of people and also their place in the society with respect to other people. Goffman (1963) used the term 'Stigma' to explain the reactions of the people to illness in society. This perspective deals with every aspect of daily life that is affected by the illness and 'degree of stigmatization'.

Gerhardt (1989) described the experience of ailing person at two levels and came up with two models to explain effects of onset of chronic diseases and then afterwards adaption to a new and changed situation by the individual. These two models are:

- Crisis Model: This model deals with the situation when a person suffers an irreversible damage physically due to some chronic disease.

- Negotiation Model: This is based on the idea of adopting a coping mechanism to live a normal life irrespective of the disability or degeneration.

Bury's work (1991) also focused on the experience of sick person at different stages of illness. He particularly dealt with the 'meanings' that go on changing in day to day interactions as a result emergence of chronic disease. Bury talks about the 'biographical disruption' i.e. physical inability to perform the task after suffering from chronic disease. This physical disability results in the loss of confidence at personal and societal level. To cope up with this disruption, a process of 'adjusting' or 'adapting' to the new conditions takes place both physically and socially. During this process of adjustment the emphasis is on positive aspects of life so as to balance and denounce the negative influence of illness.

Further, Conrad and Barker (2010) explained the development of the concept of social construction of health. They explained that reality is a social construction. It is the culture that helps in defining that which illnesses are stigmatized and considered as disabilities and which are not. Culture plays a huge role in how an individual experiences illness. It means that the illness experiences are subjective and not the objective ones and thus depend upon the individual's perceptions of it. The social construction of the illness experience deals with such issues as the way some patients control the manner in which they reveal their diseases and lifestyle adaptations they develop to cope with their illnesses. Further, medical knowledge is socially constructed; that is, it can both reflect and reproduce inequalities in gender, class, race, and ethnicity.

**Post-Modern Approach**

Post-modern theory has its origin in Post-structuralism. Post-modernism is concerned with the concept of breakup and transformation of modern society and emergence of different social conditions as compared to previously present conditions. This perspective emphasizes an increase in individualization that results in to autonomy in choosing the lifestyle and risk behavior for the individual. Thus this perspective shows a shift from structure to agency where an individual is responsible for his health rather that finding faults with social structure.

This perspective is used in few works as far as the field of medical sociology is concerned. In the present study, this perspective is useful when there is stress on personal or individual responsibility of the people's health (Cockerham, Alfred & Thomas, 1997) and preference for use of alternative system of healthcare over the existing one. (McQuaide, 2005).

**Psycho-Social Perspective**

Psycho-social perspective emphasized the role of psychological and social factors in causing a disease. According to Elstad (1998), the main reason for health disparities in affluent societies is psychological stress and the fabrication of psychological stress is embedded in the social and interpersonal ties. Thus, social and community networks as well as the stress are the determining factors in causing or preventing the diseased condition (Durkheim, 1966).

Moreover, stressful life events produce the physiological and emotional responses and are related with the onset of cancers, heart diseases, diabetes, stroke etc. (Link and Phelan, 1995). Therefore, both stress and disease have their origin in the society.

**Health Lifestyle Theory**

Cockerham (2005) explained the health lifestyle theory. The source of his theory was two main concepts specified by Max Weber and P. Bourdieu. These concepts were life chances and lifestyle choices (Weber, 1978) and the concept of habitus (Bourdieu, 1984).

In the words of Cockerham (2000a), health lifestyle is "the collective patterns of health related behaviour based on choices from options available to people according to their life chances." Here, life chances are said to be similar to social structure and lifestyle choices are as alternate to agency. Now, these lifestyle choices are enabled or constrained by the life chances i.e. social structure. Thus, social structure plays an important role by influencing the lifestyle choices and thus, chances of availing the good things in life.

Further, the life chances or structural variables like social class, age, gender, race or ethnicity, living conditions etc. determine the lifestyle choices and these lifestyle choices may be healthy or unhealthy. The healthy lifestyle includes healthy diet, physical activity etc. whereas unhealthy lifestyle is use of tobacco and alcohol, unhealthy diet etc. The people or group having similar life chances may have healthy or unhealthy lifestyle determined by the selection of their lifestyle choices.

**REVIEW OF LITERATURE**

Review of literature is an effort to know about the already existing information related to the field under study. This helps us to acquaint ourselves with the research works carried till date in the concerned field. The present study is focused on lifestyle related diseases among doctors. Since the present study falls in the domain of medical sociology, so an effort is made by the researcher to review the literature related to this topic that exists both in medical and sociological domain.

The studies in medical domain are carried primarily by community medicine and public health departments. The studies are mostly based upon quantitative data collected on the basis of surveys. The sociologists also have tried to explore various areas in medical sociology, though   most of the work is focused on various aspects of diseases and healthcare professionals. There are very few studies done so far to understand the sociological aspects of lifestyle related diseases among doctors.

## I.  Studies done in Medical Domain

Studies done in this domain are mainly related to occupational stress among doctors, their lifestyle habits, presence of lifestyle related diseases among doctors, their illness behaviour, doctor-patient relationship etc.

### *Studies related to 'Lifestyle Habits' of Doctors*

The studies on the lifestyle habits of doctors include daily activities linked to the exercise, diet, nutrition, sleep, consumption of alcohol and smoking etc. These lifestyle habits eventually may become the risk factors for causation of lifestyle related diseases. The studies by Philibert (2005); Lockley et al. (2007); Wada et al. (2011); Wiskar (2012); Jardim et al. (2015); and Hegde, Vijayakrishnan, Sasankh, Venkateswaran, Parasuraman (2016) are included in this section.

Philibert (2005) explored the effect of sleep deprivation on the cognitive and clinical performance on 959 physicians and 1028 non-physicians. The study revealed that effect of lack of sleep was more in non-physicians as compared to physicians and continuous working hours without required hours of sleep affect negatively the cognitive and clinical performance.

Lockley's (2007) study was focused on exploring the effect of working hours and sleep deprivation of healthcare workers on their safety and performance. The study came to conclusion that long working hours had adverse effect on healthcare providers leading to increase in fatigue related medical and diagnostic errors, occupational injuries, motor vehicle accidents. The study suggested a safe work-hour limit for the healthcare professionals.

The study by Wada et al. (2011) focused on the lifestyle habits related to diet, exercise, smoking and alcohol among doctors working at hospitals in Japan. The study revealed prevalence of lack of exercise was the highest and smoking was the lowest as far as these four lifestyle habits were concerned. The study stressed the need for awareness about health among doctors.

Wiskar (2012) studied the issues related to nutrition, exercise, sleep and self-care among doctors. The study suggested that like common man physicians should also improve their lifestyle related behavior by taking healthy and nutritious diet, proper sleep and exercise because health of the physicians is closely related to the well-being of patients and in providing quality healthcare to them.

Jardim et al. (2015) explored the prevalence of risk factors for cardio-vascular diseases in different areas of health care such as pharmacology, odontology, nursing, medicine and nutrition department over a period of 20 years. The study highlighted that despite having knowledge about the risk factors still there is presence of a large number of risk factors like sedentary lifestyle, alcohol consumption, overweight, dyslipidemia responsible for cardiac-vascular diseases among health care professionals.

Cross-sectional study among 250 doctors and nurses in a medical college hospital in Tamil Nadu was done by Hegde et al. (2016) with an objective of knowing about the lifestyle associated risk factors for cardio-vascular diseases among doctors and nurses. The study revealed that doctors are at higher risk of cardio-vascular diseases as compared to nurses and general population.

***Studies related to 'Occupational Stress' Among Doctors***

Some studies had been done to recognize the job related stress among doctors. For instance, studies by Menon & Munalula (2007); Wond (2008); Huggard & Dixon (2011); Govender, Mutunzi & Okonta (2012) and Tuthill, Ahmed, Mathewe, Balton & Molokhia (2013).

Menon and Munalula (2007) examined the job related stress among doctors. For this purpose, a pilot study had been done with a sample of forty one doctors with in an age group of 24-43 years and with a working duration of eight months to nineteen years in University Teaching Hospital, Lusaka, Zambia. The study recoganized a large numbers of stressor like excessive work load, stressful long duty hours, financial problems, conflict between personal and professional life etc. which are detrimental to physical and mental health of doctors.

Wond's article (2008) observed the job related stress among doctors because of the excessive demands linked to their work. The article discussed the sources and consequences of stress and barriers in availing the healthcare services. The study suggested some preventive measures to deal with the stress.

Huggard and Dixon (2011) carried out study with a sample of 253 doctors with different areas of specialization working at four locations in New Zealand. The study concluded that experience associated with compassion fatigue in doctors is similar to that of other healthcare professionals like social workers, counselors, psychologists and nurses. The study concluded that one in six doctors is at the risk of compassion fatigue and one in five doctors is having the danger of burn out.

Govender et al. (2012) studied stress among doctors of all age groups working in four public hospitals of Ngaka Modiri Molema, N-W province of South Africa and concluded that work related stress among doctors is more than the general working population. The study suggested that doctors need to take active measures to reduce their stress.

The article by Tuthill et al. (2013) focused on the work associated stress among doctors working in University Hospital Lewisham and came to the conclusion that medical profession is the most stressful one. There is no significant difference in stress levels between different grades of doctors such as doctors working in intensive care unit and medicine as well as an anesthetist.

***Studies related to 'Lifestyle related Diseases' Among Doctors***

There are very small number of studies i.e. studies by Lin S-Y et al. (2013); Kim et al. (2016) and Purohit and Verma (2016) that explored the presence of chronic diseases among doctors.

Lin S-Y et al. (2013) carried out a study of cohort of 22,309 physicians in Taiwan and found that physicians are at lower risk of cancer as compared to general population. The risk of thyroid, prostrate, breast and non-cervical gynecological cancer is higher among physician as compared to general population. Further, the overall cancer rate among female physicians is higher than the male physicians.

The study by Kim et al. (2016) is based on the health examination of 382 doctors at a health examination center between 2010-2013. The study revealed high prevalence of cancer incidence among doctors in Korea as compared to general population. The most commonly found cancer among male doctors is that of stomach and thyroid cancer whereas among female doctors,  breast, cervix and lung cancer are the most common ones.

The Study by Purohit and Verma (2016) revealed the prevalence of non-communicable diseases in doctors due to their faulty lifestyle. Doctors have to work under stressful conditions. They also do not have an adequate sleeping hours due to their work schedule. Due to such type of hectic daily routine, they are unable to follow a healthy lifestyle like regular diet pattern and physical work out that leads to obesity, cardiovascular disease, diabetes and hypertension. Also, to deal with the stress they develop the habit of consumption of alcohol and tobacco that manifest in to development of cancer and respiratory problems.  Though doctors are considered to be the learned segment of the society yet due to their unhealthy lifestyle they suffer from non-communicable diseases.

### *Studies related to 'Illness Behavior' of Doctors*

The studies related to illness behaviour of doctors include the experiences of doctors as patients, habit of self-medication among doctors, barriers perceived by doctors in taking treatment etc.

Few studies such as studies by Turner and Brian (2000); Gautam and MacDonald (2001); Jaye and Wilson (2003) dealt with experiences of doctors as patients, their behaviour during illness etc.

Turner and Brian (2000) talked about the emotional dimensions of chronic diseases due to difficulty in adjustments with the changed lifestyle and long term treatment which is commonly overlooked. This emotional trauma leads to development of depression and anxiety among such sufferers. The study suggested the psycho-social aspects of care along with medical care to cope up the situation.

Gautam and MacDonald (2001) talked about the prevalence of chronic illness among physicians, challenges faced by 'doctor-patient' and physician of 'doctor-patient' and suggestions to deal with their chronic diseases. Doctors always have a denial attitude in accepting the illness and management of disease is difficult for them. The study suggested the comprehensive approach at the personal and professional level to cope up with the chronic conditions for the doctors.

Jaye and Wilson (2003) work dealt with the experience of illness by GPs (General practitioners), the change they had felt towards themselves and towards the treatment of their patients. It also discussed the barriers faced by GPs in consulting some other physicians. Due to this health needs of GPs were seriously compromised because of attitudes toward illness with in medical profession. This study also talked about self-referral and self-prescription. This study threw light on the role ambiguity faced by physician and 'doctor-patient' at two different levels i.e. at the level of doctor of a 'doctor-patient' and as a 'doctor-patient'.

Another studies such as studies by Mckevitt & Morgan (1997); Thompson, Cupples, Sibbert, Skan & Bradley (2001); Kay, Michell & Del (2004); Kay, Clavarino, Doust & Jenny (2008) and Garelick (2012) explored the barriers faced by doctors in seeking treatment during illness.

Mckevitt & Morgan (1997) explored main barriers in healthcare seeking behavior of doctors. This study was conducted with an interview of 64 doctors who had been suffering from physical and mental illness. A sense of stigma was present in case of mental illness and a feeling of guilt and embarrassment were present both in case of acute and chronic physical illness. Denial of being sick was the main barrier in availing the health care services.

A study by Thompson et al. (2001) throws light on the barrier experienced by the general practitioner as a result of their attitudes of self-denial, stigma and embarrassment about illness and concern about the confidentiality of the illness. This study recommended that medical education, training and culture should strive to promote appropriate health care among doctors.

The study by Kay et al. (2004) revealed limited availability of data on the physical well-being of practitioners. Doctors ignore the issues related to their physical health. They neither go for preventive health measures nor do they have personal general practitioners.

The study by Kay et al. (2008) is based on analysis of 26 articles having information related to barriers faced by doctors while accessing the healthcare services. Health care access of doctors fall into three categories- Do doctors have their doctors, do doctors go to the doctors or they take self treatment. According to this study, near about all the doctors are registered with general practitioner. Almost all the doctors go for self-treatment for minor illnesses. Self treatment was more common for general practitioner (GP) than specialists. The paper discussed the barriers at different levels like patient, provider, system and cultural level.

Garelick in his study (2012) revealed the barriers faced by the doctors in accessing the health care services. This study recommends a clear strategy to regulate health care services in the form of specialist services for doctors. Specialist services should be holistic in approach focusing on the individual health needs of the patient, balancing the professional and personal life and clinical and organizational issues at work.

Few studies i.e. studies by Laskari et al. (2010); Montgomery (2011); Schulz et al. (2016) focused the habit of self treatment among doctors.

Laskari et al. (2010) found that a huge number of doctors are self-prescribing due to medical knowledge and accessibility of prescribed medicines. The reasons behind the self-medication were a feeling of being stigmatized, lack of time to visit a doctor and to avoid sick leave during illness.

The study by Montgomery (2011) was review of twenty seven studies conducted from 1990-2009. It revealed that most of the studies reported self-medication for both acute and chronic treatment. The main reasons for self-medication were avoiding the role of patient, acceptance of self-treatment as a norm, work performance or pressure to remain at work and confidentiality to keep the things within one's control or in a small number of chosen colleagues.

Schulz et al. (2016) found that only one fifth doctors were registered with GPs. More than half of the doctors had one chronic condition. The study pointed towards the high rates of self-treatment especially in case of acute diseases. Respondents with chronic conditions and working in collective practices were more likely to be registered with GP. Main barrier in seeking help were lack of time and non-availability of local GP.

*Studies related to Doctor-Patient Relationship*

Some other studies by Ferguson and Candib (2002); Wong and Lee (2006); Ha and Longnecker (2010); DeBenedette (2011); Mahato and Suman (2013) focused on the doctor-patient relationship.

The study by Ferguson and Candib (2002) was based on the review of twenty one articles and the studies in these articles were categorized into language barrier studies, bias studies on the part of doctors and studies on doctor-patient relationship. The study concluded that race, ethnicity and language play an important role in the quality of doctor-patient relationship.

Wong and Lee (2006) explored the role of communication skill in doctor-patient relationship. According to them, better doctor-patient communication results into better physical, mental, and emotional health and decreasing the illness symptoms, better improvement in chronic conditions like controlled blood pressure and sugar level.

The study by Ha and Longnecker (2010) revealed the importance of effective communication between doctor and patient in providing the good health care. The study also talked about the barriers in good and skilled communication on both doctor and patient side. The study recommends the training of doctors in inter-communication skills.

DeBenedette (2011) observed the factors responsible for better engagement of patient in healthcare such as good communication between doctor-patient, patient's perception about doctor's behavior as respectful, patient-physician communication outside the scheduled working hours i.e. informal communication.

The main objective of the study by Mahato and Suman (2013) is to assess status of doctor-patient relationship in clinical practice and enhanced awareness among clinicians in this regard. This study concluded that most of the doctors agreed that good doctor-patient relationship helps in good and effective treatment outcome.

## II. Studies Done in Sociological Domain

Studies in sociological domain are done in department of sociology and department of sociology and anthropology. Most of the studies primarily carried in Indian context took into consideration the structural aspect of medical profession and different systems of medicine. There are few studies available on illness behavior of patients in chronic diseases and doctor-patient relationship.

*Sociological Studies related to 'Illness Behaviour' in Chronic Illnessess*

Malathi (1993); Mukund (2002); Prabakar (2010); Ray (2011); Achidambaranathan (2011); Babu P (2017) focused on illness behaviour of the people in the chronic diseases like diabetes, cancer, hypertension, heart diseases in their research works .

The research work by Malathi (1993) discussed the social epidemiology and illness behaviour among the females suffering from cancer of cervix. This study tried to explore the pre-diagnostic and post-diagnostic illness behaviour of the females suffering from chronic illness like cancer of cervix. The study revealed that incidence of cancer are common among the women belonging to different age groups, previous history of cancer was missing among majority of cases and majority of women were in the third stage of cancer. The study found that status inconsistency as the major cause for stress among the women that consequently was the main cause for cancer among women. The risk factors like nature of menstruation and personal and menstrual hygiene depended upon the education, literacy among females etc. Perception and evaluation of symptoms were influenced by the cultural factors and socio-economic status. A feeling of social isolation, alienation, powerlessness and normlessness had also been observed.

The study by Mukund (2002) focused on the perceptions and expectations as well as the problems faced by the people suffering from heart diseases and by their caretakers. It was found that males were more vulnerable to development of heart diseases and stress was the major factor for causation of these diseases. All the aspects of life were affected by the heart diseases. Socio-psychological impacts were more visible than the economic impact. An improvement of relationship between spouses as well as between parents and children had been observed. Majority of respondents felt no affect on their social life. Positive role played by religion and family in coping up the psychological impact i.e. fear, anxiety and stress etc. had been reported.

Prabakar (2010) studied the problems faced by people suffering from chronic diseases. The study concluded that the people find it difficult to adjust with social relationships. The study revealed that after 2006 there was a shift in trend in the development of diseases. Now, these diseases were more common among females and were mostly found among the persons above 50 years of age. The people also found it hard to manage the normal social, outdoor and household activities. Psychological impact of disease such as anxiety, fear etc. had also been felt as a result of occurrence of these diseases. Due to increase in the dependency on the family members, a tension in the social relationships had been observed. The study suggested that prevention of these diseases should be preferred and programs should be specifically designed to address this issue.

Ray (2011) explored the awareness level and access of treatment by the cancer patients in West Bengal. The study revealed that literate people were more aware about this disease as compared to illiterate ones. Unawareness also persisted regarding the infectious or non-infectious nature and symptoms of cancer. The people having awareness about the hospitals treating cancer patients were 63.20%. Lower awareness level about the treatment was found among the people with lower socio-economic and educational status and from rural background. The attitude of the family members was also found to be compassionate with such patients. Very small number of patients (6.20%) was willing to hide their diseased condition from neighbors or outsiders. Majority of patients (69.50%) were not aware about the risk factors associated with the cancer. Participation in cancer awareness programme and awareness about the government relief fund was observed among small number of patients. Prevalence of cancer was more common among females and in rural areas. Stage 3 of cancer was more frequently found among low income group and illiterate. Presence of health facility at far off place and money were the main constraints in taking treatment. Early detection of cancer was more observed in educated, high income group and in urban areas.

The study by Achidambaranathan (2011) was carried in four villages i.e. two coastal and two inland villages of Tirunelveli district of Tamilnadu to analyze the relationship between the social practices of the village folk and their diseases. The study found that prevalence of chronic diseases (35.80%) was higher than the acute diseases (25.45%) among people of these four villages. The percentage of people with no health problem was 38.80%. The percentage of people  suffering from chronic cases in coastal villages  (45%) was found to be higher as compared to the people of inland villages (31.30%). In case of acute diseases, prevalence among respondents of inland village (29.60%) was more than their counterparts in coastal village (17%). The study also found that religious offerings, home remedies, prayers and socio-religious beliefs were followed by the people for the treatment of their diseases.

The study by Babu P (2017) is focused upon the adjustments with the diabetes by the diabetic patients. The study supported that there was not much social impact of diabetes on the people suffering from diabetes. Adaptation level was found to be directly related to the educational level as well as the income of the diabetics. Also, adaptation level was better among employed as compared to unemployed. Difference between the adaptation levels of male and female and people residing in the nuclear and joint family was observed to be significant. The variations in knowledge and perception for treatment, quality of life, economic strains etc. among the diabetic patients were influenced by the occupations, education status, religions, marital status etc.

***Sociological Studies related to Doctor-Patient Relationship***

The studies by Carstairs (1955); Minocha (1974); Hasan (1979); Srivastva (1979); Advani (1980); Tiwari (1999) are mainly focused on the doctor-patient relationship.

The study by Carstairs (1955) was carried in two villages of Rajasthan i.e. in Sujarupa and Delwara has revealed the perceptions of the physician and the village people about reasons behind development of disease and methods of curing.  According to him, rural people perceive that the origin of diseases is celestial in nature and rooted in human conduct. The illness is considered as moral as well as physical crisis. So they try to get relief from the ailing condition with the help of rituals and home remedies. The acceptance of modern system of medicine can only be possible if a relationship of  faith develops between the sufferer and the healer. This faith can be established only if there is slow spread of information about the infections and technology. Also, understanding the perspective of patients when they approach the doctors for treatment was key to establish trust between doctors and patients. The study highlights the problems in developing the mutual trust between doctor and patient because both have the different perceptions about illness and for methods of treatment because of their different cultural background.

The study by Minocha (1974) was done in Lady Harding Medical College, New Delhi. For the present study, the sample consisted of only female patients. The embedded aim of the study was to understand the perspective of female patient for modern medicine. The study revealed that development of modern medicine affected the nature of doctor-patient relationship. The advancement in modern medicine like specialization in particular field of medical stream resulted in alterations of role of doctors and thus, the role of doctors became impersonal. Also, there are a number of cultural barriers that affect the interaction between doctors and patients and consequently act as deciding factors for the suitable treatment of patients. In the study, it was also found that most of the female patients discontinue the treatment and stay in the hospital against the advice of doctors. The reasons may be the inability of patients to afford the treatment as it is expensive or there may be the chances of lack of communication between the doctor and patient because the Indian women being introverted communicate with male doctors through their male family members or care takers. The study suggested that acceptance of modernization in the domain of health and illness would felicitate the adjustment to the modernization in other domain.

The case study presented by Hassan (1979) in his book on 'Medical Sociology and Rural India' focused upon the relationship between doctor and patient in a village setup. The study revealed that rural people were more comfortable while discussing their health related issues with the folk medical practitioners as compared to practitioners from modern medicine. They had more trust in folk medical healers whereas a sense of  suspicion and fear prevailed while visiting a modern medical practitioner. Moreover, villagers were used to have free medical consultation and folk medicine, so they found it difficult to spend money on medicine and consultation in case of physicians practicing modern medicine. He reported that physician was consulted for the treatment only when either the etiology of diseases was not clear or more advanced treatment of the disease was not accessible. Thus, this study highlighted the results of the introducing modern medicine and behavioral factors responsible for success or failure of the practitioner of modern medicine  in the village.

Srivastava's (1979) study in Sir Sunder Lal hospital in Varanasi explored the nature of interface between the doctors and para-medical staff and consequently its effect on the relationships between doctors and patients. The study found that main barriers to communication among doctors, patients and para-medical staff were lack of education and difficulty in understanding the language. There was big gap between role expectations and role performance by the doctors. The findings of the study also revealed that cultural norms play an important role while addressing the problem of health and illness and both administrative structure and working in the hospital was influenced by these norms. Besides, interaction between doctors and patients was affected by their socio-cultural status rather than socio-economic status of patients. The doctors wanted to have a formal relationship with the patients whereas patients expected an informal and close interaction. Too much administrative control and lack of appreciation for abilities of the working professionals were the big reasons for the disagreement in the hospital.

Advani (1980) discussed 'Doctor-patients relationship in Indian hospital' and highlighted the role expectations from doctors and patients in their respective statuses. He found that practice of doctors was influenced by their social status and professional ethics. Doctor should not only be polite and sympathetic with their patients but also provide the moral support to the patient during treatment. Doctor should instruct the patient about the healthy diet and preventive measures to be taken to avoid the diseases and further deterioration of health. On the other hand, patients should cooperate during treatment, they should be brief, specific and frank while explaining their health related problem to doctors.

The other findings of the study were- professional satisfaction of doctors was directly related whereas the quality of doctor-patient relationship was inversely connected to the size of the hospital. Socio-economic status of the patients affects the choice of the type of hospital i.e. private or government hospital.

The study by Tiwari (1999) discussed the effectiveness, accessibility and impact of different systems of medicine like Allopathy, Ayurvedic, Unanai and Homeopathy as well as doctor-patient relationship in these systems. The study revealed that as the doctors are from high and middle income groups, so it becomes difficult for them to relate with the poor rural masses. Despite the popularity of Allopathy system of medicine for treatment, the indigenous systems of medicine are still influential as far as the treatment is concerned. No major difference in behaviour of doctors belonging to different systems of medicine has been observed in terms of number of patients diagnosed per day or dealing with patients. Doctors in private hospital are more cordial towards patients as compared to doctors working in government hospital. Doctors working in Allopathy hospitals have formal interaction with patients in comparison to doctors working in Homeopathy, Ayurvedic and Unani hospitals. Relationship between doctors and patients are affected by mother tongue, socio-economic status, profession of patients etc. Social and community networks play an important role in the selection of systems of medicine, doctors and treatment procedure for treatment. Besides, in India, people spend their savings for the medical treatment.

***Studies related to 'Structural Aspect' of Medical Profession***

Madan (1972, 1980);    Mathur (1975); T.K.Oomen (1978); Ramanamma & Bambewale (1978); Venkatarathnam (1979); Ambica Chandani (1980);    Kumar (1986); Madhu Nagla (1990) ; Abidi (1992); Minocha (1996) discussed structural aspects of medical profession like the role structures of doctors and nurses, role expectations, role performance, role conflict, personality traits of doctors etc.

Two studies by Madan (1972, 1980) i.e. "Doctors in a north Indian city: Recruitment, role perception and role performance " and "Doctors and Society" were carried in two different domains. The first study was related to private practitioners and was focused on "who are the doctors in terms of their social background, how and why they have been trained, and how they related themselves to their work, and implicitly or explicitly to society." The second study was concerned with the doctors practicing at the All India Institute of Medical Sciences, Delhi. In this study, three main issues related to doctors were addressed. The first was-how the doctors perceive and understand their role as doctors, how they evaluate the place where they were working and how they relate themselves with the society in which they work and live.

The studies found that doctors are only technically qualified and they are unaware about the prevailing social and cultural setup of the society. They are primarily concerned with their educational upgradation for their own gain. With such kind of mindset, they either emigrate to foreign countries or they prefer to serve the affluent people. Their success is related to their professional competence and technical skill rather than goodwill. This analysis brings out the different aspects of doctors' personality in medical profession.

The study by Mathur (1975) was done in a hospital which was connected to a medical college situated in Rajasthan. The main focus of the study was on the human organization involving interpersonal relationships among the various strata of medical staff as well as with patients. The study revealed that hospital was a subsystem of a larger system i.e. medical college.

The conformist and non-conformist behaviour in this hospital was influenced by not only the internal organization of subsystem such as hospital but also by the organization of the medical college. The functioning of the hospital is the reflection of the socio-cultural values present in the main system i.e. in medical college. The physical and social environment in the hospital had significant effect on the treatment and recovery of patients.

Oommen (1978) carried his study in public hospitals in Delhi. The focus of this study was to examine the role structures associated with occupation of Allopathic doctors and nurses. The study focused on the change of the occupational roles of doctors and nurses when they shift from private institutions to public institutions and its effect on their working. He tried to understand the meaning of profession from the angle of ideal type construct of profession and actuality of profession.

In this study, particular areas of interests were role perceptions and role commitments of professionals, role conflict, role behavior of medical professionals, relation between social structure and profession etc. The study suggested doctors have high prestige as compared to nurses due to their social background.

Ramanamma and Bambawale (1978) highlighted the working practices of three types of doctors. These doctors were general practitioners or physicians, consultants and paid physicians. The working practices or occupational attitude was determined on the basis of time spent by doctors on patients, level of interaction between doctors and patients etc. The study observed that general practitioners were concerned about both mental and emotional healing along with the physical curing of patients whereas consultants were not much concerned about emotional and psychological well-being because they spent very less time on patients. Though paid physicians were not getting much monetary gain yet they felt satisfied by curing the patients with complicated health issues. The study concluded that these three types of practitioners had their own ways of practice, but one thing was common among them i.e. all of three types of practitioners observe the affective neutrality with the patients. The maximum level of interaction was found to be between general physicians and their patients whereas consultants and paid physicians had minimum level of interaction with their patients.

The study by Venkatratnam (1979) is related to the analysis of role of doctors and nurses in a hospital set up in Tamil Nadu. The focus of his study was mainly to analyze the role expectations and actual role performance of doctors and nurses related to their respective statuses. He used the structural-functional perspective for this purpose. The study revealed that there were different role expectations attached to the status of doctors and nurses. These role expectations and role performance were not only for their own respective statues but also from each other's statues. The study concluded that role of nurses was subordinate to that of doctors and was quasi-independent. The study also mentioned the dissatisfaction of nurses with the role performed by the doctors.

Chandani (1980) carried her study with a sample of 152 doctors in Jodhpur. In this study, she interviewed 119 institutional doctors and 33 doctors from private institutions. This study is an attempt to examine the important aspects of medical profession like motivation behind joining this noble profession, role expectations attached to the status of doctors etc. The study revealed that doctors were not interested in working in rural areas because of lack of facilities there. The doctors also prefered to do the private practice. Moreover, the medicine as a profession was decided by the family and altruism was said to be the main driving force for the selection of this profession. Humanitarian attitude, devotion and politeness should be the main qualities of medical professional but doctors are lacking these traits nowadays.

Kumar (1986) focused on the study of medical profession. The study observed that Medical Council of India (MCI) is under the control of state rather than an autonomous body and has to abide by Indian Medical Council Act. In the absence of active participation of government, MCI feels helpless. Doctors feel comfortable in working near their place of origin because of their cultural acquaintance. Moreover, parents prefer medical carrier for their children because of high socio-economic status despite the expensiveness of medical education. The discrepancy between the ideal role and actual role performance of doctors has been observed in this study. Doctors were also found to be passive for the activities such as elections of Indian Medical Association.

The study by Nagla (1990) was carried out among doctors in Medical College and Hospital, Rohtak, in Haryana. Here, she tried to find the fundamental features of profession so as to differentiate it from occupation. For this purpose, she selected the medical profession and tried to explain phenomenon of professional functioning in one of the complex institutions such as hospital. She talked about importance of medical profession in the society as well as the problems faced by doctors. Medical profession was found to be dominated by men of higher caste and class. It was found that doctors were satisfied with their profession to a large extent despite having some difficulties in practicing this profession. The reasons enlisted for dissatisfaction and frustration at work were odd and long working hours, low financial gain, lack of freedom to move etc.

Abidi (1992) carried out a study in government hospitals of Delhi to observe both social and occupational roles as well as role conflict among female doctors. While discussing the social role conflict the study found that female doctors in the status of wife and mother managed their roles of caring children, household work etc. very efficiently. No major role conflict was observed between personal and professional life. At professional front, the study revealed that role conflict was mostly visible among senior doctors as compared to junior doctors because senior doctors were more burdened with the responsibilities and their accountability was also more. The study suggested that this role conflict can be minimized if roles are managed properly.

The study by Minocha (1996) is a qualitative study of a women's general hospital in New Delhi. This study has been mentioned in her book 'Perceptions and interactions in a medical setting: A Sociological study of women's hospital'. The study describes the status and role of women associated with medical domain. The various roles related to women in hospital settings may be that of doctors, nurses, para-medical staff, as administrators or also as patients.  Further, study explains the role of caste in shaping the behaviour and stances of people during social interaction in the hospital, role played by the social obligations in solidifying the relationships during illness, people's perception and response to the advanced technological equipments like thermometer, x-rays, stethoscope etc., perception and presentation of roles by the medical and para-medical staff. The study also pointed out the dehumanizing factors prevailing in the hospital setting like non-compassionate attitude of the hospital staff, difficulties faced by the patients for admitting in the hospital, long waiting queues  in the hospitals for treatment etc.

***Studies related to 'Utilization of Different Systems of Medicine'***

The studies by Marriot (1955), Bhardwaj (1975); Joshi (1979); Jaisal (1982); Mishra (1994); Velankanni (2014) examined the preference for different systems of medicine by patients for treatment, perspectives of doctors belonging to different systems of medicine etc.

The study by Marriot (1955) explored the socio-cultural constraints in using the modern medical techniques among conservative rural folk in the Indian village of Kishan Garghi in western Uttar Pardesh. The study was focused on the social organization of the village with particular focus on the medical institutions. Here, analysis of role of western medical institutions in comparison to indigenous medical institutions from the perspective of social organization was done. The study revealed many differences and disagreements among the medical practitioners practicing two different systems of medicines i.e. indigenous and western systems of medicines. These differences and disagreements were observed in the methods of dispensing medicines and dealing with their patients. These conflicts impeded the spread of western medicines among the rural folk of western Uttar Pardesh. The author has the opinion that western medicine can successfully establish itself among the rural folk by enculturation of certain folk values and dissociating itself from some western cultural values.

The study by Bhardwaj (1975) discussed preference of people of four selected villages of Ropar district in Punjab for the type of medical practitioners practicing different systems of medicine during treatment. For this purpose, a sample of 104 households was taken to interview the heads of the households. In contrast to common belief of social scientists, the rural people of all caste groups in these villages preferred allopathic system of medicine in comparison to indigenous system of medicine. All the caste group either upper or lower castes showed significant preference for allopathic medicines whereas only four percent of the villagers in the sample opted for desi medicine. Further, approximately one third of the people said that their preference for the medicines depended upon the nature of their health problem. This suggests that recovery from disease was found to be more important than the commitment to traditional system of medicine. Not even a single physician practicing solely Ayurvadic or Unani system of medicine was found in the four villages under study.

The study by Joshi (1979) is an attempt to analyze the beliefs, attitudes and values of the people with respect to health and illness in an Indian town. The findings of the study refuted the general assumption that belief in supernatural cause and magical cure of diseases existed only in rural areas and uneducated section of the urban areas. People residing in the urban areas also had faith in the supernatural cause as well as preference for alternative system of medicine other than modern medicine for treatment. Even doctors practicing in these areas were well aware about the behaviour pattern of the people which included switching form one system of medicine to another or use of more than one system of medicine simultaneously or shifting from one doctor to another for treatment etc. The study suggested that it is necessary to understand the cultural factors in order to take the preventive measures for diseases and also indigenous system of medicine should be incorporated along with the modern system of medicine for treatment.

Research work carried by Jaisal (1982) is not the field study of disease and treatment in the society. This study is based on review of literature with some specific objectives related to medical profession i.e. doctors, patients and paramedical staff. The main objectives of the study were to find out the problems and perspectives as well as overview of medical sociology in India, international perspectives related to doctor-patient relationship and an insight in to social structure and disease in the villages of India. The study observed the dichotomy of folk medicine and modern medicine as far as the treatment of diseases in Indian villages were concerned. The study suggested an ethno-methodological approach to the medical profession because societies are not homogenous. Medical sociology was found to be in its nascent stage in India and studies so far mentioned in this research work were exploratory in nature, so, further research was recommended in medical sociology.

The study "Doctors and their professional world view: A study of Ayurvedic and Allopathic Doctors in the city of Varanasi" was carried out by Mishra (1994). This study explored the perspectives of doctors belonging to two different systems of medicine i.e. Allopathic and Ayurvedic. These perspectives were related to a number of issues such as reason behind joining the medical profession, the difference in approach for prescribing the medicine, their attitude towards patients while treating them, their participation in seminars and conferences for professional growth etc.

Velankanni (2014) made an attempt to analyze the utilization of different systems of medicine, sociological aspects of sickness, doctor-patient relationship etc. The study revealed that government hospitals were not preferred for treatment by the people, the most commonly used medicine was Allopathy followed by Homeopathy, Ayurvedic and Unani. Majority of respondents had family doctors for treatment. The doctor residing close to the respondent's house was mostly preferred. Caste was not considered important in the selection of family doctor. Most of the respondents did not practice the self-medication because they were aware of the dangerous effect of self-medication.

**RESEARCH GAPS**

From the review of literature discussed above the following research gaps were identified:

- Few studies done on lifestyle related diseases amongst medical fraternity are mainly focused on the one or the other aspect of these diseases and therefore lacks a holistic approach to understand lifestyle related diseases among doctors. Moreover, the studies are mostly done by medical professional with very little emphasis on socio-cultural aspects of these diseases.

- In sociological domain, most of the studies done so far on medical profession and doctors have focused on organizational aspects such as doctor-patient relationship, doctor's perceptions about their profession, comparison of different systems of medicines, role performance and role expectations of doctors etc. Researcher did not come across any study analyzing the social causes and consequences of lifestyle related diseases among doctors.

**SIGNIFICANCE OF STUDY**

The statistics given so far presents a grim situation related to lifestyle related diseases. This study will help in understanding the gravity of lifestyle related diseases among common people by studying the situation in a profession which is assumed to be the least affected profession as far as lifestyle related diseases are concerned.

In addition, the present study is focused upon the health condition of doctors in relation to lifestyle related diseases because if health of the healthcare provider is not good then it will become difficult for him to provide the quality care to the consumer. The study will also highlight the socio-economic and psychological aspects of lifestyle related diseases among doctors. Besides, the suggestions given for medical professionals as well as for the common people will be helpful for future planning and implementation of policies to curb the deadly growth of these diseases.

**RESEARCH QUESTIONS**

- Whether the doctors themselves have same or high degree of risk related to the presence of lifestyle related diseases as the common people? If yes, what are the reasons for prevalence of lifestyle related diseases among doctors?

- What are the risk factors associated with lifestyle related diseases?

- What is difference in lifestyle of healthy and unhealthy doctors?

- What is the social, psychological and economic impact of lifestyle related diseases on doctors?

- What are the experiences of 'doctors as patients' and physician of 'doctor-patient'?

- What are the coping strategies followed by 'doctors as patients' of lifestyle related diseases?

- What measures should be taken to curb these diseases?

**HYPOTHESIS**

- Most of doctors suffer from lifestyle related diseases.

- Doctors generally ignore the risk factors leading to lifestyle related diseases.

- Lifestyle of healthy doctors is different from the lifestyle of unhealthy doctors.

- Doctors mostly do self medication.

- Doctors are not untouched by the socio-economic and psychological effect of lifestyle related diseases.

- Doctors efficiently cope with the lifestyle related diseases.

**OBJECTIVES OF THE STUDY**

- To prepare a socio-demographic, economic and professional profile of the respondents and to find out the incidence and type of lifestyle related diseases among doctors in Punjab.

- To identify the risk factors leading to lifestyle related diseases among the doctors.

- To compare the lifestyle of healthy and unhealthy doctors.

- To examine the socio-psychological and economic impact of lifestyle related diseases on the respondents.

- To enlist the experiences of 'doctors as patients' and physician of 'doctor-patient' and to know about the coping mechanisms of respondents to tackle these diseases and their impact.

- To provide suggestions for lowering the incidence of the lifestyle related diseases among people in general and doctors in particular.

**METHODOLOGY**

Punjab was selected as universe of the present study. The reason for selection was the presence of high morbidity rate in Punjab as compared to the national average (NSSO, 2006). Further, within Punjab, the research work was carried out among doctors in two Cities of Punjab i.e. Amritsar and Patiala. These cities were selected  because the morbidity was at its minimum level in Amritsar District and at its maximum level in Patiala District as per National Sample Survey Organization data, 2004 (as cited in Swaran Singh, 2013).  The districts were thus selected on the basis of purposive sampling.

The major lifestyle changes are expected in the urban centres. For this purpose of selection of doctors, the district wise Indian Medical Association's (IMA) list of doctors had been referred. Since the number of doctors in Amritsar and Patiala were 700 and 500 respectively in Indian Medical Association list of doctors. Hence 20% of the doctors had been selected as sample from each city. Thus, a sample of 240 doctors was studied for the present study.

For the present study, purposive sampling technique was used in order to give representation to doctors from private or government sector and different areas of specialization.

The data collection was based on both Primary and Secondary methods of data collection. The Primary data was collected with the help of Interview Schedule which included the questions related to lifestyle related diseases and their risk factors, impact of these diseases on respondents, experiences of respondents as being patient, coping mechanism adopted by them etc.

In addition, a total of 17 case studies of the doctors were taken. A Focused Group Discussion of 12 doctors was also organized to have a deeper insight into the issue under study. The secondary data has been collected with the help of research articles, studies and reports by institutions of national and international repute such as National Sample Survey Organization (NSSO), National Commission on Macro-economics of Health, Step-wise Survey of Punjab (2014-2015) by PGIMER, World Health Organization (WHO) etc.

**CHAPTER SCHEME**

The first chapter dealt with introduction to the present study, statement of problem, theoretical framework, review of literature, research gaps, significance of the study, research questions, hypothesis, objectives, and methodology.

The second chapter focused on the socio-demographic, economic and professional profile and the incidence of lifestyle related diseases among the respondents.

The third chapter mentioned the socio-demographic, economic and professional profile of healthy and unhealthy doctors.

The fourth chapter compared the lifestyle and risk factors between healthy and unhealthy respondents.

The fifth chapter examined the impact of lifestyle related diseases on doctors.

The sixth chapter discussed the experiences and coping mechanism adopted by doctors suffering from lifestyle related diseases.

The seventh chapter contained Case Studies and Focused Group Discussion.

The last or eight chapter included the main findings and observations of the study as well as the suggestions for doctors to prevent and cope up with the lifestyle related diseases.

# CHAPTER II

# THE PROFILE OF THE RESPONDENTS & THE INCIDENCE OF LIFESTYLE RELATED DISEASES

It is considered that lifestyle of an individual is an outcome of the economic, social and professional position in society. This profile of the respondents can help in understanding the causes and consequences of lifestyle related diseases. Also, it is important to know the state of lifestyle related diseases among the respondents.

For the study of lifestyle related diseases among doctors in Punjab, a total sample of 240 respondents was taken from the two cities of Punjab i.e. Patiala and Amritsar. The sample included 100 doctors from the Patiala city and 140 doctors from Amritsar city. The respondents were purposively selected from the private and public domain as well as from different areas of specialization.

This chapter is divided into two sections. The first section of the chapter focuses on the socio-demographic, economic, and professional profile of the respondents. The second section describes the incidence of lifestyle related diseases among respondents.

**I**

The profile of the respondents has been further sub-divided into two parts for better description of the data. Part A deals with the socio-demographic and economic profile and Part B is concerned with the professional profile of respondents.

## A. SOCIO-DEMOGRAPHIC AND ECONOMIC PROFILE

The socio-demographic and economic profile of respondents is based upon the information related to age, gender, religion, domicile, marital status, type of family structure, and income etc.

### Age

The age is often considered important for knowing the health status of an individual. It may not only influence the lifestyle of the individuals but also sometimes acts as

45

catalyst for the occurrence of diseases. So, it is important to be familiar with the age of respondents. It helps us to find out age groups of respondents present in our sample and consequently can facilitate us in identifying the possibility of having chronic health issues among different age groups.

**Table 2.1 Distribution of Respondents on the Basis of Age (in Years)**

| City | Age (in Years) | | | | | Total |
|------|-------|-------|-------|-------|----------|-------|
|      | 31-40 | 41-50 | 51-60 | 61-70 | Above 71 |       |
| Patiala | 21(21.00%) | 31(31.00%) | 23 (23.00%) | 19 (19.00%) | 6 (6.00%) | 100 (41.67%) |
| Amritsar | 32 (22.85%) | 47 (33.57%) | 45 (32.14%) | 9 (6.43%) | 7 (5.00%) | 140 (58.33%) |
| Total | 53 (22.08%) | 78 (32.50%) | 68 (28.33%) | 28(11.67%) | 13 (5.42%) | 240 (100%) |

Table 2.1 shows that the present sample had respondents from different age groups including young, middle and old age groups. Out of 100 respondents from Patiala city, 31 (31%) were in the age group of 41-50 years and 23 (23%) were in the age group of 51-60 years. Further, 21 (21%) respondents fall in the age group of 31-40 years. Other 19 (19%) respondents were in the age group of 61-70 years and rest 6 (6%) were in the age group of above 71 years.

Out of total 140 respondents in Amritsar, 47 (33.57%) were in the age group of 41-50 years and 45 (32.14%) in the age group of 51-60 years. Other 32 (22.85%) fall in the age group of 31-40 years and 9 (6.43%) in the age group of 61-70 years. Rest 7 (5%) respondents were in the age group of above 71.

Thus, maximum number i.e. 78 (32.50%) of respondents in both cities come in the age group of 41-50 years and minimum number of respondents i.e. 13 (5.42%) fall in the age group of above 71 years. The age of the youngest respondent was 31 years whereas that of the eldest one was of 78 years.

The data thus  show that majority (82.91%) of the respondents were in the age group of 31-60 years. Further, the age increased beyond 61 years of age, the number of respondents decreased.

This may be due to the fact that after the age of 60s many of the doctors either retire from government job and those in private practice may start refraining from the active professional life.

**Gender**

Gender may affect the lifestyle of the person and accordingly, determine the health of the people. Generally, the lifestyle of men differs from that of women. So it was desired to find out the number of male and female respondents in the selected sample.

**Table 2.2 Distribution of Respondents on the Basis of Gender**

| City | Gender | | Total |
|---|---|---|---|
| | **Male** | **Female** | |
| Patiala | 58 (58.00%) | 42 (42.00%) | 100 (41.67%) |
| Amritsar | 87 (62.14%) | 53 (37.86%) | 140 (58.33%) |
| Total | 145 (60.42%) | 95 (39.58%) | 240 (100%) |

Table 2.2 indicates the distribution of respondents on the basis of gender in both the cities of Punjab. In the total sample of 240, 145 (60.42%) were male respondents and 95 (39.58%) were female respondents. Out of total 145, male respondents, 58 belonged to Patiala city and 87 respondents were from Amritsar city. Whereas, out of total 95 females respondents, 42 and 53 female respondents were from Patiala and Amritsar respectively.

The presence of more number of male i.e. 145 (60.42%) in the selected sample may be due to the fact that men opt for medical career more as compared to women. Similarly, the study by Goodnow (1990) also revealed that science is considered as more appropriate cultural task for men as compared to women.

**Religion**

Religious beliefs, values and norms may have great effect on the lifestyle of people. Thus it was considered imperative to know religion of the respondents.

**Table 2.3 Distribution of Respondents on the Basis of Religion**

| City | Religion | | | | Total |
|---|---|---|---|---|---|
| | **Hindu** | **Sikh** | **Muslim** | **Christian** | |
| Patiala | 56 (56.00%) | 40 (40.00%) | 3 (3.00%) | 1 (1.00%) | 100 (41.67%) |
| Amritsar | 75 (53.57%) | 59 (42.14%) | 4 (2.85%) | 2 (1.42%) | 140 (58.33%) |
| Total | 131 (54.58%) | 99 (41.25%) | 7 (2.91%) | 3 (1.25%) | 240 (100%) |

Table 2.3 depicts the distribution of respondents on the basis of religion. Out of total number of 240 respondents, 131 (54.58%) respondents were from Hindu community, 99 (41.25%) were from Sikh community, 7 (2.91%) respondents were from Muslim community and only 3 (1.25%) were from Christian community.

The number of Hindu respondents was 56 (56%) in Patiala and 75 (53.57%) in Amritsar. The respondents belonging to Sikh community were 40 (40%) in Patiala and 59 (42.14%) in Amritsar city. The researcher came across only 7 (2.91%) respondents from Muslim community (3 in Patiala and 4 in Amritsar city). There were 3 (1.25%) respondents from Christian community in both the cities in the sample.

Thus, majority (95.83%) of the doctors in the sample were from both Hindu and Sikh religion in the selected cities. This may be because of the fact that the present research is based in Amritsar and Patiala cities of Punjab where the majority of population follows Sikh and Hindu religion.

**Rural-Urban Domicile**

Place of living is important in defining the lifestyle of people. Living culture and lifestyle of urban people is different from that of rural people. Urban culture shows more inclination toward the fast food consumption and sedentary as well as materialistic lifestyle. The background of the respondents was noted on the basis of their rural-urban domicile.

**Table 2.4 Distribution of Respondents on the Basis of Rural-Urban Domicile**

| City | Domicile | | Total |
|---|---|---|---|
| | **Rural** | **Urban** | |
| Patiala | 33 (33.00%) | 67 (67.00%) | 100 (41.67%) |
| Amritsar | 39 (27.86%) | 101 (72.14%) | 140 (58.33%) |
| Total | 72 (30.00%) | 168 (70.00%) | 240 (100%) |

As shown in Table 2.4, out of total 240 respondents, 72 (30%) respondents were from rural background while 168 (70%) were from urban background.

In Patiala, 33 (33%) respondents were from rural background and 67 (67%) belonged to urban areas. In Amritsar, 39 (27.86%) respondents were from rural background while 101 (72.14%) were from urban background. Thus, respondents from both urban and rural background were found in the sample.

**Marital Status**

Marital status can be vital in shaping the lifestyle of people. Lifestyle of individuals of different marital status i.e. married, unmarried, divorcee and widow/widower may be dissimilar from each other. So, it was desired to find out the marital status of respondents in our sample. This may help us to further identify the effect of marital status on the occurrence of lifestyle related diseases.

**Table 2.5 Distribution of Respondents on the Basis of Marital Status**

| City | Marital Status | | | | Total |
|---|---|---|---|---|---|
| | **Married** | **Unmarried** | **Widow/Widower** | **Divorcee** | |
| Patiala | 77 (77.00%) | 18 (18.00%) | 4 (4.00%) | 1 (1.00%) | 100 (41.67%) |
| Amritsar | 121 (86.43%) | 17 (12.14%) | 0 (0.00%) | 2 (1.43%) | 140 (58.33%) |
| Total | 198 (82.92%) | 35 (14.58%) | 4 (1.67%) | 3 (1.25%) | 240 (100%) |

Table 2.5 specifies about the marital status of the respondents. Out of 240 respondents, 198 (82.92%) were married and 35 (14.58%) were unmarried. Further, 4 (1.67%) respondents were widow/ widower and 3 (1.25%) were divorcee.

Out of 198 married respondents, 77 (77%) were from Patiala and 121 (86.43%) belonged to Amritsar. There were 18 (18%) unmarried respondents from Patiala and 17 (12.14%) unmarried respondents from Amritsar. All the 4 (4%) widow or widower respondents belonged to Patiala whereas out of total 3 (1.25%) divorcees, 1 (1%) divorcee was from Patiala and 2 (1.43%) divorcee respondents were from Amritsar

Majority (82.92%) of the respondents were married. This is probably due to the fact that all of the respondents were above the age of 30 which is a marriageable age in India.

**Type of Family Structure**

Family is often considered an important institution act as a part of social support system for an individual. The role of family during the time of crisis is very crucial. A person suffering from a long term health issue needs the help of family members to deal with the difficulties associated with onset of a chronic disease.

The knowledge about the family of respondent i.e. nuclear or joint family may help in discovering the presence of social support system.

**Table 2.6 Distribution of Respondents on the Basis of Family Structure**

| City | Family Type | | Total |
|---|---|---|---|
| | **Nuclear** | **Joint** | |
| Patiala | 57 (57.00%) | 43 (43.00%) | 100 (41.67%) |
| Amritsar | 75 (53.57%) | 65 (46.43%) | 140 (58.33%) |
| Total | 132 (55.00%) | 108 (45.00%) | 240 (100%) |

As we know that process of urbanization has propagated the culture of nuclear family structure, it is evident in our sample also. Table 2.6 highlights that out of total sample of 240 respondents, 132 (55%) were from nuclear family structure and 108 (45%) were from joint family structure.

In Patiala, out of 100 respondents, 57 (57%) belonged to nuclear family structure and 43 (43%) were from joint family structure while in Amritsar, the number of respondents from nuclear and joint family structure was 75 (53.57%) and 65 (46.43%) respectively.

Thus, the data indicate that in both the cities the number of respondents belonging to nuclear family structure was more than the respondents from joint family structure. This appears to be in line with the general trend of nuclear families in cities in Punjab.

**Income per Annum**

Economic status affects the lifestyle of the people. It is usually seen that the people belonging to the higher income groups have a rather luxurious and sedentary lifestyle. This kind of lifestyle may have a remarkable effect on the health of the people in later age. So, it is also wished to discern the annual income of respondents. It will give us the idea about the present life chances and living standards of the respondents.

**Table 2.7 Distribution of Respondents on the Basis of**

**Income per Annum (In Lacs)**

| City | Income per Annum | | | Total |
|---|---|---|---|---|
| | <10 lacs | 10-20 lacs | >20 lacs | |
| Patiala | 25 (25.00%) | 44 (44.00%) | 31 (31.00%) | 100 (41.67%) |
| Amritsar | 42 (30.00%) | 52 (37.14%) | 46 (32.85%) | 140 (58.33%) |
| Total | 67 (27.91%) | 96 (40.00%) | 77 (32.08%) | 240 (100%) |

Table 2.7 shows the income per annum of the respondents. Out of total 240 respondents, 96 (40%) fall in the range of 10-20 lacs per annum whereas 77 (32.08%) were in the income group of >20 lacs per annum and 67 (27.91%) belonged to <10 lacs per annum income group. Thus, maximum number (40%) of respondents fall in the income group of 10-20 lacs while minimum number (27.91%) of respondents were from <10 lacs annual income group.

The similar trend prevails in Patiala and Amritsar individually. The maximum number of respondents in Patiala. 44 (44%) belonged to 10-20 lacs per annum income group followed by 31 (31%) respondents from >20 lacs per annum and 25 (25%) respondents within <10 lacs per annum income group In Amritsar, 52 (37.14%) respondents fall in the income group of 10-20 lacs, 46 (32.85%) in >20 lacs and 42 (30%) belonged to <10 lacs income group.

This seems to indicate that doctors are the high earning group of society and high income propagates a luxurious lifestyle.

## B. PROFESSIONAL PROFILE OF RESPONDENTS

Professional profile of respondents encompasses the area of specialization, type of working institution, number of working days per week, number of duty hours per day etc.

### Area of Specialization

In medical profession, there are basically two branches i.e. non-clinical and clinical branches. Non-clinical branches mainly associated with teaching job in medical colleges include Anatomy, Physiology, Pharmacology, and Pathology etc. as area of specialization whereas clinical branches are directly involved in the treatment of the patients and include the specialization in Surgery, Gynecology, Pediatrics, Medicine, Skin, Orthopedics, and Eye, ENT etc. Clinical branches are considered to be busier and time demanding as compared to non-clinical branches.

It is essential to know about the area of specialization so as to be acquainted with the lifestyle of the respondents. The respondents working in clinical branches may have more hectic work schedule than the respondents working in non-clinical branches of the medical profession. This may help us to recognize the lifestyle of the respondents and later on the effect of area of specialization on health of respondents.

**Table 2.8 (a) Distribution of Respondents on the Basis of
Area of Specialization (Non-clinical Branches)**

| Non-clinical Branches | City | | Total |
|---|---|---|---|
| | Patiala | Amritsar | |
| Anatomy | 7 (25.00%) | 4 (8.88%) | 11 (15.06%) |
| Physiology | 3 (10.71%) | 4 (8.88%) | 7 (9.58%) |
| Pharmacology | 8 (28.57%) | 8 (17.77%) | 16 (21.91%) |
| SPM* | 1 (3.57%) | 7 (15.56%) | 8 (10.95%) |
| Pathology | 6 (21.42%) | 9 (20.00%) | 15 (20.54%) |
| Microbiology | 0 (0.00%) | 5 (11.11%) | 5 (6.84%) |
| Forensic | 2 (7.14%) | 4 (8.88%) | 6 (8.21%) |
| Biochemistry | 1 (3.57%) | 4 (8.88%) | 5 (6.84%) |
| Total | 28 (38.35%) | 45 (61.64%) | 73 (100%) |

*SPM- Social and Preventive Medicine

Table 2.8 (a) specifies that out of 73 respondents from non-clinical branches, 16 (21.91%) respondents were from Pharmacology, 15 (20.54%) from Pathology, 11 (15.06%) belonged to Anatomy and 8 respondents (10.95%) were from SPM. Other 7 (9.58%) belonged to Physiology and 6 (8.21%) respondents were from Forensic. Rest 5 (6.84%) respondents were from Microbiology and 5 (6.84%) from Biochemistry. Within non-clinical branches, maximum numbers i.e. 16 (21.91%) were in Pharmacology and minimum numbers of respondents were in Biochemistry and Microbiology i.e. 5 (6.84%).

**Table 2.8 (b) Distribution of Respondents on the Basis of**

**Area of Specialization (Clinical Branches)**

| Clinical Branches | City | | Total |
| --- | --- | --- | --- |
| | Patiala | Amritsar | |
| Surgery | 14 (19.44%) | 13 (13.68%) | 27 (16.16%) |
| Skin | 5 (6.94%) | 1 (1.05%) | 6 (3.59%) |
| Orthopedics | 5 (6.94%) | 11 (11.57%) | 16 (9.58%) |
| Medicine | 17 (23.61%) | 33 (34.73%) | 50 (29.94%) |
| Pediatrics | 0 (0.00%) | 4 (4.21%) | 4 (2.39%) |
| Gynaecology | 11 (15.27%) | 17 (17.89%) | 28 (16.76%) |
| Eye | 9 (12.5%) | 2 (2.10%) | 11 (6.58%) |
| ENT* | 3 (4.16%) | 5 (5.26%) | 8 (4.79%) |
| Psychiatry | 5 (6.94%) | 3 (3.15%) | 8 (4.79%) |
| Radiotherapy | 3 (4.16%) | 1 (1.05%) | 4 (2.39%) |
| Anesthesia | 1 (1.38%) | 4 (4.21%) | 5 (2.99%) |
| Total | 72 (43.11%) | 95 (56.88%) | 167 (100%) |

*ENT- Ear, Nose and Trachea

Table 2.8 (b) shows that out of 167 respondents from clinical branches, 50 (29.94%) respondents were from Medicine, 28 (16.76%) from Gynecology and 27 (16.16%) from Surgery. Other 16 (9.58%) respondents were from Orthopedics, 11 (6.58%) respondents were Eye specialist, 8 (4.79%) were ENT specialist and 8 (4.79%) respondents were Psychiatrist. Rest 6 (3.59%) respondents were Skin specialist, 5

(2.99%) respondents were from Anesthesia, 4 (2.39%) respondents belonged to Pediatrics and 4 (2.39%) were Radiotherapist. Within the clinical branches, maximum number of respondents i.e. 50 (29.94%) in the sample was from Medicine branch of specialization and minimum numbers of respondents i.e. 4 (2.39%) were from Pediatrics and Radiotherapy branch of specialization.

Thus, Table 2.8 (a) and (b) indicate that out of total 240 respondents, 73 (30.41%) respondents were from non-clinical branches and 167 (69.58%) respondents were from clinical branches and thus, large numbers of respondents 167 (69.58%) were from clinical branches of medical profession.

**Type of Working Institution**

Work culture of private institution may be different from the work culture of government institution. It is generally assumed that work pressure in private sector is much more than the work pressure in public sector. Thus knowing about the type of working institution of the respondents may help in determining the lifestyle of the respondents and therefore, effect of the lifestyle on the health of the respondents.

**Table 2.9 Distribution of Respondents on the Basis of Type of Working Institution**

| City | Working Institution | | Total |
| --- | --- | --- | --- |
| | Private | Public | |
| Patiala | 38 (38.00%) | 62 (62.00%) | 100 (41.67%) |
| Amritsar | 29 (20.71%) | 111 (79.28%) | 140 (58.33%) |
| Total | 67 (27.91%) | 173 (72.08%) | 240 (100%) |

Table 2.9 shows that out of 240 total respondents, 173 (72.08%) were working in Public institutions and 67 (27.91%) were in Private institutions. In Patiala, 38 (38%) respondents were in Private institutions and 62 (62%) were in Public institutions. In Amritsar, 29 (20.71%) respondents were working in Private and 111 (79.28%) in Public institutions.

Majority of the respondents in our sample i.e. 173 (72.08%) were working in public or government institutions.

**Nature of Job**

Nature of job may affect the daily routine of the people. The respondents associated with teaching in medical college and working only in OPD may have more relaxed daily routine than the respondents working in both OPD and IPD. Hectic daily routine may affect not only the eating and sleeping habits of the people but may also be detrimental for the health of the people.

In the present study, the researcher wanted to know the effect of nature of job on the lifestyle and accordingly on the health of the respondents. So, it was desired to identify the number of respondents in different areas of job whether OPD, IPD, both OPD and IPD or teaching in the selected sample.

**Table 2.10 Distribution of Respondents on the Basis of Nature of Job**

| City | Nature of Job | | | | Total |
|---|---|---|---|---|---|
| | **OPD*** | **IPD**** | **Both** | **Teaching** | |
| Patiala | 21 (21.00%) | 1 (1.00%) | 57 (57.00%) | 21(21.00%) | 100 (41.67%) |
| Amritsar | 27 (19.28%) | 4 (2.85%) | 89 (63.57%) | 20 (14.28%) | 140 (58.33%) |
| Total | 48 (20.00%) | 5 (2.08%) | 146 (60.83%) | 41(17.08%) | 240 (100%) |

*OPD- Out Door Patients    **IPD- In Door Patients

As shown in Table 2.10, out of total number of 240 respondents, number of respondents working in both OPD and IPD was 146 (60.83%), 48 (20%) respondents were working in OPD only, 41 (17.08%) in teaching and 5 (2.08%) were working in IPD. In Patiala, 57 (57%) respondents were working in both OPD and IPD, 21 (21%) were working in OPD and 21 (21%) were in teaching and 1 (1%) worked in IPD. In Amritsar city, 89 (63.57%) respondents worked in both OPD and IPD, 27 (19.28%) were in OPD, 20 (14.28%) were in teaching and 4 (2.85%) respondents were working in IPD.

Maximum number of respondents i.e. 146 (60.83%) were working in both OPD and IPD and least number of respondents 5 (2.08%) were working in IPD.

Here, it is imperative to know that teaching subjects are related to non-clinical branches of medical profession. Generally, the doctors specialized in non-clinical branches either teach in medical colleges or they do the job/practice where there is no direct interaction with the patients. But researcher in this study came across some respondents though specialized in non-clinical branches but involved in practice like specialist in clinical branches, so these respondents were counted under OPD type of job/practice.

**Experience of Medical Practice**

Lifestyle of individuals may vary according to the number of years put by them in the profession. In the initial years of the career, the doctors have to work day and night to earn name and fame. Due to this work schedule, they may have a hectic and demanding life which may later on affect the health of an individual. So, the researcher was interested to know the duration of professional practice/job of the respondents.

**Table 2.11 Distribution of Respondents on the Basis of**

**Years of Medical Practice**

| City | Years of Medical Practice | | | | | | Total |
|---|---|---|---|---|---|---|---|
| | 0-10 | 11-20 | 21-30 | 31-40 | 41-50 | Above 50 | |
| Patiala | 22 (22.00%) | 32 (32.00%) | 16 (16.00%) | 24 (24.00%) | 5 (5.00%) | 1 (1.00%) | 100 (41.67%) |
| Amritsar | 26 (18.57%) | 37 (26.42%) | 48 (34.28%) | 17 (12.14%) | 10 (7.14%) | 2 (1.42%) | 140 (58.33%) |
| Total | 48 (20.00%) | 69 (28.75%) | 64 (26.67%) | 41 (17.08%) | 15 (6.25%) | 3 (1.25%) | 240 (100%) |

The Table 2.11 depicts that out of total 240 respondents, 69 (28.75%) were in practice for 11-20 years, 64 (26.67%) were for 21-30 years and 48 (20%) respondents were for 0-10 years. Other 41 (17.08%) respondents were in practice for 31-40 years, 15 (6.25%) were for 41-50 years and 3 (1.25%) were in practice for more than 50 years.

In Patiala, out of 100 respondents, 32 (32%) respondents were in medical practice for 11-20 years, 24 (24%) were for 31-40 years, 22 (22%) were for 0-10 years, 16 (16%) were for 21-30 years, 5 (5%) were in practice for 41-50 years and there was only 1(1%) respondent working for more than 50 years.

In Amritsar, out of total 140 respondents, 48 (34.28%) were in practice for 21-30 years, 37 (26.42%) for 11-20 years, 26 (18.57%) for 0-10 years, 17 (12.14%) were for

31-40 years, 10 (7.14%) respondents were for 41-50 years and there were 2 (1.42%) respondents whose experience of practice was above 50 years.

From the above data, it is clear that most of the respondents i.e. 222 (92.50%) were having an experience of up to 40 years of medical practice and least number of respondents i.e. 18 (7.50%) were in practice for more than 40 years.

**Number of Working Days per Week**

Number of working days in a week tells about the work schedule of the respondents. A full week work schedule without any break may result in to busy daily schedule that may have harmful effect on the health of respondents. So, question was asked from respondents related to number of working days per week.

**Table 2.12 Distribution of Respondents on the Basis of Number of Working Days per Week**

| City | Working Days per Week | | Total |
|---|---|---|---|
| | **7 Days** | **< 7 Days** | |
| Patiala | 27 (27.00%) | 73 (73.00%) | 100 (41.67%) |
| Amritsar | 66 (47.14%) | 74 (52.85%) | 140 (58.33%) |
| Total | 93 (38.75%) | 147 (61.25%) | 240 (100%) |

Table 2.12 indicates that out of total sample of 240 respondents, 147 (61.25%) were working less than 7 days a week while 93 (38.75%) were working 7 days a week. Out of total 147 (61.25%) respondents working less than seven days a week, 73 (73%) were from Patiala and 74 (52.85%) were from Amritsar city whereas out of total 93 (38.75%) respondents working 7 days a week, 27 (27%) belonged to Patiala and 66 (47.14%) were from Amritsar.

Importantly, 93 (38.75%) respondents in our sample said that they worked all the seven days a week without any break.

**Number of Duty Hours per Day**

Number of duty hours per day reveals about the work load of the respondent. If the duty hours are less and fixed, it may result in to more relaxed and streamlined daily routine but if the duty hours 'depend upon the situation' it may cause relatively irregular and stressful daily routine. So, number of duty hours per day may help in to be familiar with the daily routine of the respondent and thus, its effect on the health of respondents.

Table 2.13 Distribution of Respondents on the Basis of Number<br>of Duty Hours per Day

| City | Daily Working Hours | | | Total |
|------|------|------|------|-------|
| | >8 Hours | <8 hours | Depends Upon Situation | |
| Patiala | 22 (22.00%) | 38 (38.00%) | 40 (40.00%) | 100 (41.67%) |
| Amritsar | 57 (40.71%) | 37 (26.42%) | 46 (32.85%) | 140 (58.33%) |
| Total | 79 (32.91%) | 75 (31.25%) | 86 (35.83%) | 240 (100%) |

Table 2.13 shows that out of total sample of 240 respondents, 86 (35.83%) respondents' daily working hours 'depends upon the situation' at the work place, 79 (32.91%) respondents worked more than 8 hours in a day and 75 (31.25%) respondents did the work for less than 8 hours a day.

In Patiala, maximum numbers of respondents i.e. 40 (40%) respondents' working hours 'depend upon situation' and 38 (38%) respondents worked < 8 hours a day and 22 (22%) respondents were working >8 hours a day. In Amritsar, maximum numbers of respondents i.e. 57 (40.71%) were working > 8 hours a day, 46 (32.85%) respondents' work 'depend upon situation' and 37 (26.42%) respondents worked < 8 hours a day.

From the above data, it appears that respondents in the category where working hours 'depend upon the situation' were ready to work for > 8 hours a day. Thus more numbers of respondents i.e. 165 (68.75%) were working for long hours in a day.

**II**

**INCIDENCE AND TYPE OF LIFESTYLE RELATED DISEASES**

In this section, primarily incidence i.e. number of respondents affected by lifestyle related diseases and type of lifestyle related diseases such as hypertension, diabetes, respiratory diseases, heart problem, cancer etc. have been discussed. Also, we have tried to describe the information associated with the duration of disease, perceived reasons behind disease, presence or absence of family history of disease etc.

**Presence/Absence of Lifestyle related Diseases**

Presence or absence of a disease tells about the state of physical wellbeing of an individual. So, question was asked whether the respondents had some type of lifestyle related disease.

**Table 2.14 Distribution of Respondents on the Basis of Presence/Absence of**

**Lifestyle related Diseases**

| City | Presence of Lifestyle related Diseases | | Total |
| --- | --- | --- | --- |
| | Yes | No | |
| Patiala | 55 (55.00%) | 45 (45.00%) | 100 (41.67%) |
| Amritsar | 75 (53.57%) | 65 (46.42%) | 140 (58.33%) |
| Total | 130 (54.16%) | 110 (45.83%) | 240 (100%) |

Data in the Table 2.14 show that out of 240 respondents, 55 (55%) from Patiala and 75 (53.57%) from Amritsar were having some kind of chronic disease and 45 (45%) from Patiala and 65 (46.42%) from Amritsar had no chronic illness.

Thus, data indicate that more than half of respondents (54.16%) were suffering from lifestyle related diseases.

**Type of Lifestyle related Disease**

There are different types of lifestyle related diseases such as hypertension, arthritis, diabetes, cardiac problem, cancer etc. Question was asked from 130 unhealthy respondents about the type or types of lifestyle related diseases they were suffering from.

**Table 2.15 Distribution of Respondents on the Basis of Type of**

**Lifestyle related Diseases**

| Lifestyle related Disease | City | | Total* |
|---|---|---|---|
| | **Patiala** | **Amritsar** | |
| Hypertension | 39/55 | 34/75 | 73 (56.15%) |
| Diabetes | 13/55 | 21/75 | 34 (26.15%) |
| Asthma | 1/55 | 3/75 | 4 (3.07%) |
| COPD (chronic obstructive pulmonary disease) | 0/55 | 0/75 | 0 (0.00%) |
| Other lung diseases | 0/55 | 0/75 | 0 (0.00%) |
| Heart disease | 4/55 | 9/75 | 13 (10.00%) |
| Arthritis | 7/55 | 3/75 | 10 (7.69%) |
| Cancer | 0/55 | 3/75 | 3 (2.30%) |
| Other chronic conditions (spondylitis, thyroid, immune system problem etc.) | 15/55 | 20/75 | 35 (26.92%) |

*Multiple Responses

From Table 2.15 it is clear that the unhealthy respondents were suffering from more than one lifestyle related disease. Data in the above Table depict that 73 (56.15%) respondents were hypertensive, 35 (26.92%) respondents were suffering from other chronic diseases like spondylitis, thyroid, immune system problem etc. , 34 (26.15%) respondents were diabetic and 13 (10%) respondents were suffering from heart problem. Further, 10 (7.69%) respondents had arthritis, 4 (3.07%) respondents had asthma and 3 (2.30%) respondents were suffering from cancer. There was no respondent suffering from COPD and other lung diseases among 130 unhealthy respondents.

The data tell that maximum number i.e. 73 (56.15%) were suffering from hypertension and least number of respondents were suffering from cancer i.e. 3 (2.30%) respondents.

Hence, this finding seems to be in consonance with the findings of Global Status Report on non-communicable diseases (WHO, 2014) that reveals that in India, every tenth person is having raised blood glucose level and every fourth person aged 18 years or above has raised blood pressure levels. Thus, estimating high incidence of lifestyle related diseases in India.

Similarly, the study by Purohit and Verma (2016) also mentioned the prevalence of chronic non-communicable diseases among doctors. However, study by Kim et al. (2016) in Korea does not go with the findings of present research because their study revealed high prevalence of cancer incidence among doctors in Korea as compared to general population while in the present data there were only 3 (2.30%) respondents suffering from cancer out of total 130 unhealthy respondents.

**Perceived Reasons for Lifestyle related Diseases**

As already said lifestyle related disease is caused by faulty lifestyle of an individual and lifestyle of one individual may differ from another. There can be a number of reasons responsible for the onset of lifestyle related diseases. These reasons become the risk factors for the causation of disease. So, in order to know the prevalence of risk factors among 130 unhealthy respondents it was desired to recognize the respondents' perception of reasons for lifestyle related diseases.

**Table 2.16 Distribution of Respondents' Perception of Reasons for**

**Lifestyle related Diseases**

| City | Reasons for Lifestyle related Diseases | | | | |
|---|---|---|---|---|---|
| | **Stress** | **Lack of Exercise** | **Alcohol and tobacco consumption** | **Unhealthy Diet** | **Other factors** |
| Patiala | 36/55 | 14/55 | 13/55 | 10/55 | 9/55 |
| Amritsar | 61/75 | 21/75 | 9/75 | 11/75 | 5/75 |
| Total* | 97(74.61%) | 35(26.92%) | 22 (16.92%) | 21 (16.15%) | 14(10.76%) |

*Multiple Responses

Table 2.16 indicates more than one reason given by respondents for development of their chronic conditions. There were 97 (74.61%) respondents who said that their ailing condition was due to stress, 35 (26.92%) felt lack of exercise as the reason and 22 (16.92%)  respondents perceived consumption of alcohol/tobacco as the main cause for their disease. Moreover, 21 (16.15%) told unhealthy diet as the reason and rest 14 (10.76%) respondents assigned other reasons like age factor, heredity as possible cause responsible for lifestyle related diseases.

Thus, from the above findings, it is clear that doctors perceived that they had many risk factors like stress, unhealthy diet, lack of exercise etc. Out of these risk factors one or more than one may be the reasons for their diseased condition.

In many Case Studies i.e. 001 to 005, respondents mentioned unhealthy lifestyle and in Cases 006 to 010, stress has been assigned as the main reason for the development of lifestyle related diseases.

The above findings can be related to the various studies on unhealthy lifestyle among doctors, for instance, studies related to 'lifestyle habits' of doctors by Wada et al. (2011), Wiskar (2012), Jardim et.al  (2015), Hegde et al.  (2016) highlighted the presence of risk factors such as sedentary lifestyle, overweight, sleep deprivation, physical inactivity, alcohol taking, tobacco use, unhealthy diet etc. among doctors. These risk factors may lead to development of lifestyle related diseases.

The data in our study show that the doctors were aware that they were having risk factors which may cause one or more lifestyle related diseases.

**Diagnosis of Disease for the First Time**

Diagnosis means 'detection of a disease' which is a preliminary step for starting treatment. It is usually seen that common people get them diagnosed only on the appearance of symptoms in their body. Here, we wanted to make out that how the doctors came to detect their chronic illness for the first time.

**Table 2.17 Distribution of Respondents on the Basis of the Diagnosis of Disease**

| City | Diagnosis of Disease | | Total |
|---|---|---|---|
| | **During Routine Check-ups** | **Symptoms Appeared** | |
| Patiala | 22 (40.00%) | 33 (60.00%) | 55 (42.30%) |
| Amritsar | 28 (37.33%) | 47(62.67%) | 75 (57.69%) |
| Total | 50 (38.46%) | 80 (61.53%) | 130 (100%) |

Table 2.17 shows that out of 130 unhealthy respondents, 80 (61.53%) got their disease diagnosed after the appearance of symptoms and 50 (38.46%) respondents came to know about their illness during routine health check-ups.

This shows that majority of respondents i.e. 80 (61.53%) came to know about their illness only after appearance of symptoms. This points towards the callousness of doctors to undergo the routine medical examination.

In Cases 001 and 005, doctors came to know about their chronic illness i.e. diabetes only after the appearance of symptoms.

This finding can be related to the findings by Kay et al. (2004) which revealed that doctors ignore the issues related to their physical health. They neither go for preventive health measures like routine medical check-ups nor do they have personal general practitioners.

**History of Illness**

History of illness tells that for how many years the person is suffering from the disease. If a person is suffering from lifestyle related diseases since a long period of time, then the person may be more susceptible to development of complications of lifestyle related diseases. To know this, question was asked from the 130 unhealthy respondents about the duration of illness.

**Table 2.18 Distribution of Respondents on the Basis of History of Illness**

| City | History of Illness (in Years) | | | | Total |
|---|---|---|---|---|---|
| | **0-10** | **11-20** | **21-30** | **>30** | |
| Patiala | 34 (61.81%) | 10 (18.18%) | 7 (12.72%) | 4 (7.27%) | 55 (42.30%) |
| Amritsar | 54 (72.00%) | 14 (18.67%) | 4 (5.33%) | 3 (4.00%) | 75 (57.69%) |
| Total | 88 (67.69%) | 24 (18.46%) | 11 (8.46%) | 7 (5.38%) | 130 (100%) |

As shown in the Table 2.18, history of illness was 0-10 years in 88 (67.69%) respondents and 11-20 years in 24 (18.46%) respondents. Further, history of illness was 21-30 years in 11 (8.46%) respondents and > 30 years in 7 (5.38%) respondents.

The data show that maximum numbers of respondents i.e. 88 (67.69%) were suffering from illness for 0-10 years while minimum numbers of respondents i.e. 7 (5.38%) had diseased condition for more than 30 years.

This data indicate that unhealthy respondents having the shortest history of illness (up to 10 years) were maximum (67.69%) and unhealthy respondents having the longest history of illness (more than 30 years) were minimum (5.38%) in number. It appears that incidence of these diseases has increased in recent times due to invasion of modern and westernized culture.

**Family History of Disease**

Family history can also be a cause for the occurrence of a disease along with the faulty lifestyle of the people. So while discussing about lifestyle related diseases it is imperative to know about the presence of family history of a disease among all the 240 respondents in the sample.

**Table 2.19 Distribution of Respondents on the Basis of Presence/Absence of**

**Family History of Lifestyle related Disease**

| City | Family History of Disease | | Total |
|---|---|---|---|
| | **Yes** | **No** | |
| Patiala | 60 (60.00%) | 40 (40.00%) | 100 (41.67%) |
| Amritsar | 85 (60.71%) | 55 (39.28%) | 140 (58.33%) |
| Total | 145 (60.41%) | 95 (39.58%) | 240 (100%) |

Data in the Table 2.19 show that out 145 (60.41%) respondents having family history of one or the other lifestyle related disease, 60 (60%) from Patiala and 85 (60.71%) from Amritsar. In all 95 (39.58%) respondents had no family history of the disease. ( 40 (40%) from Patiala and 55 (39.28%) from Amritsar )

The data indicate that more number of respondents i.e. 145 (60.41%) were having family history of disease. As said earlier, the doctors suffering from lifestyle related diseases were 130 (54.16%) while the family history of disease was present in 145 (60.41%) respondents. This shows that reason behind causation of disease may not always be genetic and lifestyle plays an important role for the development of a disease.

**Type of Family History of Disease**

There are a number of lifestyle related diseases e.g. diabetes, hypertension, heart diseases, arthritis, hypertension, respiratory disease etc. As already mentioned, there were 145 respondents with a family history of lifestyle related diseases. Researcher was further interested to identify the type of lifestyle related disease prevailing in the family of respondents. This would help in knowing the effect of genetic factor in occurrence of lifestyle related diseases.

**Table 2.20 Distribution of Respondents on the Basis of Type of**

**Family History of Disease**

| Type of Disease | City | | Total* |
|---|---|---|---|
| | Patiala | Amritsar | |
| Hypertension | 43/60 | 48/85 | 91 (62.75%) |
| Diabetes | 31/60 | 42/85 | 73 (50.34%) |
| Asthma | 0/60 | 3/85 | 3 (2.06%) |
| COPD | 0/60 | 0/85 | 0 (0.00%) |
| Other lung diseases | 0/60 | 0/85 | 0 (0.00%) |
| Heart disease | 5/60 | 9/85 | 14 (9.65%) |
| Arthritis | 3/60 | 3/85 | 6 (4.13%) |
| Cancer | 1/60 | 3/85 | 4 (2.75%) |
| Other chronic Conditions | 3/60 | 3/85 | 6 (4.13%) |

* Multiple Responses

Data in the Table 2.20 show that out of total 145 respondents with a family history of one or the other lifestyle related disease, 91 (62.75%) respondents had family history of hypertension, 73 (50.34%) respondents had family history of diabetes, and 14 (9.65%) respondents had family history of heart disease. Moreover, 6 (4.13%) respondents had family history of arthritis and 6 (4.13%) respondents had family history of other chronic conditions. Other, 4 (2.75%) respondents were having family history of cancer and 3 (2.06%) respondents having family history of asthma, and there was no (0%) respondent having family history of COPD and other lung diseases.

Further, from the data of family history and the type of disease the respondents had, we came to know that family history of hypertension was reported by 91 respondents but actual number of respondents suffering from hypertension was 73. Further, 73 respondents had family history of diabetes but actually only 34 respondents were diabetic. Similarly, for other diseases also the number of respondents actually suffering from lifestyle related diseases in our sample was less than the number of respondents having the family history of same disease. This shows that as per general notion, heredity may not be the sole reason for the causation of diseases. There may be other reasons related to day to day life that play a considerable role for the causation of disease.

**SUMMARY**

Socio-demographic, economic and professional profile of the respondents has been discussed in this chapter. The data revealed information related to age, gender, religion, rural-urban background, marital status, type of family structure i.e. nuclear or joint, income per annum of the respondents, area of specialization, number of working days and hours etc.

As far as the age was concerned, majority of the respondents (83%) fall in the age group of 31-60 years. The number of male respondents (60.42%) was more as compared to the female respondents (39.58%). Religion wise both Hindu (54.58%) and Sikhs (41.25%) were there in the sample. Majority (70%) of the respondents were from urban background. Due influence of urbanization, the number of respondents belonging to nuclear family structure (55%) was more in number as compared to respondents from joint family structure (45%). Majority (82.92%) of the respondents were married as compared to unmarried (14.58%), widow or widower (1.67%) and divorcee (1.25%). As far as the income per annum was concerned 40% of respondents earned between 10-20 lacs, 32.08% got >20 lacs and rest 27.91% had <10 lacs income per annum.

Professional profile showed that respondents from both the clinical and non-clinical branches of medical field were present in the sample. The profile revealed that among the clinical branches of medical field, maximum numbers of respondents were from Medicine branch (29.94%) of specialization and least were from Radiotherapy (2.39%) and Pediatrics (2.39%) branches of specialization. Whereas in non-clinical branches, maximum number of respondents were from Pharmacology (21.91%) and minimum number were from Biochemistry (6.84%) and Microbiology (6.84%) domain.

Majority (72.08%) of the respondents were working in the government hospitals as compared to private institutions (27.91%). Maximum (60.83%) number of respondents were working in both OPD and IPD and minimum (2.08%) number of respondents were in IPD. Professional experience of majority of the respondents was up to 50 years and a significant number (38.75%) of respondents were working a full week without any vacation. The working hours of the respondents (32.91%) also crossed the limit of 8 hours per day that revealed the hectic and long duration work schedule of the respondents.

As far as the status of health among the respondents was concerned, 130 (54.16%) out of total 240 respondents had one or another type of lifestyle related disease. Hypertension (73) and diabetes (34) were the most common disease amongst the respondents. Around 100 respondents with lifestyle diseases highlighted stress as the main cause. Most (61.53%) of the respondents came to know about their disease only after the symptoms appeared rather than in routine medical check-ups (38.46%). Further, most (67.69%) of the respondents had history of illness up to 10 years whereas there were few respondents (5.38%) with the history of disease for more than 30 years.

Also, data showed that although 60.41% respondents out of total 240 had family history of disease but 54.16% respondents had lifestyle related diseases. This shows that genetics may not be the only cause for development of lifestyle related diseases. Lifestyle also plays a significant role.

Finally, the information collected from the chapter provided a deeper insight into various aspects of the respondents. The socio-demographic, economic and professional profiles and state of lifestyle related diseases among the doctors provided a concrete foundation to proceed the study in right direction.

## CHAPTER III

## SOCIO-DEMOGRAPHIC, ECONOMIC AND PROFESSIONAL PROFILE  OF THE HEALTHY AND UNHEALTHY DOCTORS: A COMPARISON

In the previous chapter, we noted the profile of the respondents.  However, it is important to find out the similarities and differences in the profile of the healthy and unhealthy doctors in the sample. This comparison can help us to understand the differences in vulnerability of the respondents belonging to different profiles as far as the lifestyle related diseases are concerned.

In the present chapter, a comparison of the profiles of healthy and unhealthy respondents has been made. The comparison has been divided in two parts. In first section, socio-demographic and economic profile of healthy and unhealthy respondents has been compared and in second section, professional profile of respondents is taken into consideration for comparison.

As highlighted in the previous chapter, out of total sample of 240 respondents there are 110 healthy and 130 unhealthy respondents.

I

**SOCIO-DEMOGRAPHIC AND ECONOMIC PROFILE**

Socio-demographic and economic profile includes information about the age, gender, domicile, religion, family structure, marital status, income etc. of the respondents.

**Age**

Aging is defined as, "A progressive and generalized impairment of function resulting in a loss of adaptive response to stress and in a growing risk of age-associated disease" (Kirkwood, 1963). Thus, age may be a deciding factor for the good health of an individual. Since the lifestyle related diseases are also known as the 'Diseases of Longevity', so incidence of these diseases may increase as the age advances.

To know about the age of healthy and unhealthy respondents is essential because it helps to know the age group that is most and least affected by lifestyle related

69

diseases. Further, the trend in number of healthy and unhealthy respondents can be determined as the age advances.

**Table 3.1 Distribution of Healthy/Unhealthy Respondents on the Basis of Age (in Years)**

| Age (in Years) | Health Status | | Total |
| --- | --- | --- | --- |
| | Healthy | Unhealthy | |
| 31-40 | 35 (66.03%) | 18 (33.96%) | 53 (22.08%) |
| 41-50 | 41 (52.56%) | 37 (47.43%) | 78 (32.50%) |
| 51-60 | 27 (39.70%) | 41 (60.29%) | 68 (28.33%) |
| 61-70 | 6 (21.42%) | 22 (78.57%) | 28 (11.67%) |
| Above 70 | 1 (7.69%) | 12 (92.30%) | 13 (5.42%) |
| Total | 110 (45.53%) | 130 (54.17%) | 240 (100%) |

Above Table 3.1 shows the distribution of healthy and unhealthy respondents agewise. In the age group of 41-50 years, there were 41 (52.56%) healthy and 37 (47.43%) unhealthy respondents Number of healthy and unhealthy respondents were 35 (66.03%) and 18 (33.96%) respectively in the age group of 31-40 years. Further, there were 27 (39.70%) healthy and 41 (60.29%) unhealthy respondents in age group 51-60 years. There were 6 (21.42%) healthy and 22 (78.57%) unhealthy respondents in the age group 61-70 years and 1 (7.69%) healthy and 12 (92.30%) unhealthy respondents were found in age group of above 70 years.

The data indicates that maximum number of healthy respondents i.e. 41 out of 110 fall in age group of 41-50 years and maximum number of unhealthy respondents i.e. 41 out of 130 was in age group of 51-60 years.

Further, it is also clear from the above data that the number of unhealthy respondents increased with the increase in age of the respondents. Up to 40 years of age there was almost double number of healthy respondents i.e. 35 (66.03%) as compared to unhealthy respondents 18 (33.96%) but in the age group of 41-50 years, there is not much difference in the number of healthy (41) and unhealthy (37) respondents. After the age of 50 years, the number of unhealthy respondents showed an upward trend as compared to healthy respondents. Thus, data in Table 3.1 point towards the fact that lifestyle related diseases are the 'Diseases of longevity'.

It is relevant to mention here the study by Prabakar (2010) where higher occurrence of chronic diseases have been discussed among the people above 50 years of age.

However, in contrast to the above quantitative data, the various case studies gave mixed results. For example, in Case Study 006 cardiac problem developed at the young age of 28 years whereas in Case Study 010 doctor suffered from rheumatoid arthritis at very young age of 35 years. Also, Case Studies 002, 003, and 016 cannot be related to the above findings where doctors reported that they developed hypertension at a very young age of 18, 24, and 35 years respectively.

Importantly, Case nos. 011, 012, 013 reported to be healthy even after the age of 50 years. Thus, we could find several cases which show that nowadays age is not the sole criteria for the development of lifestyle related diseases.

During the Focused Group Discussion, this was the general view point that incidence of lifestyle related diseases increases with the advancement of age but most of the participants were also of the opinion that despite popular as 'diseases of longevity', these diseases are currently being quite common in the younger generation also.

**Gender**

Jovicic (2015) and Vari et al. (2016) after analyzing the high risk behaviors concluded that various types of healthy and unhealthy behaviors among men and women are promoted by gender behaviors and attitudes. Gender related behaviors may affect the health of an individual.

Distribution of healthy/unhealthy respondents on the basis of gender helps us to know about gender that is more vulnerable to lifestyle related diseases as compared to the other.

**Table 3.2 Distribution of Healthy/Unhealthy Respondents on**

**the Basis of Gender**

| Gender | Health Status | | Total |
|---|---|---|---|
| | **Healthy** | **Unhealthy** | |
| Male | 59 (40.68%) | 86 (59.31%) | 145 (60.42%) |
| Female | 51 (53.68%) | 44 (46.31%) | 95 (39.58%) |
| Total | 110 (45.83%) | 130 (54.17%) | 240 (100%) |

The data in Table 3.2 show that out of total 145 (60.42%) male respondents, 59 (40.68%) were healthy and 86 (59.31%) were unhealthy whereas out of 95 (39.58%) female respondents, 51 (53.68%) were healthy and 44 (46.31%) were unhealthy.

Among unhealthy respondents, the number of male respondents i.e. 86 was almost double as compared to female respondents i.e. 44. So, it appears that men are more vulnerable to lifestyle related diseases as compared to women.

Similarly, Mukund (2002) while studying the incidence of heart diseases among people observed that men are more vulnerable to these diseases as compared to women.

**Religion**

Religion often influences the culture and lifestyle of the individuals. The religion wise distribution of healthy and unhealthy respondents helps us to identify the religion with maximum and minimum number of healthy and unhealthy respondents.

**Table 3.3 Distribution of Healthy/Unhealthy Respondents**

**on the Basis of Religion**

| Religion | Health Status | | Total |
|---|---|---|---|
| | **Healthy** | **Unhealthy** | |
| Hindu | 56 (42.75%) | 75 (57.25%) | 131 (54.58%) |
| Sikh | 47 (47.47%) | 52 (52.53%) | 99 (41.25%) |
| Muslim | 5 (71.43%) | 2 (28.57%) | 7 (2.91%) |
| Christian | 2 (66.67%) | 1 (33.33%) | 3 (1.25%) |
| Total | 110 (45.83%) | 130 (54.17%) | 240 (100%) |

Table 3.3 indicates that out of total 240 respondents, 131 (54.58%) were Hindus, 99 (41.25%) were Sikhs, 7 (2.91%) were Muslims and 3 (1.25%) were Christians. Among unhealthy respondents, majority i.e. 75 (57.25%) out of total 131 came from Hindu community, followed by Sikh community i.e. 52 (52.53%) out of total 99. There is lesser number of unhealthy respondents reported from Muslim community i.e. 2 (28.57%) out of total 7 and Christian community i.e. 1 (33.33%) out of 3.

The data highlights that among all the respondents, respondents belonging to all the communities in Punjab carry good number of unhealthy as well as healthy respondents. Though the Muslims and Christians were carrying lesser percentage of unhealthy respondents which may be due to their smaller number in the sample.

**Rural-Urban Domicile**

Physical and mental health of an individual not only depends upon the 'way of living' but also the 'place of living'. Place of living can be seen as a container that involves physical, social and cultural components (Fitzpatrick & LaGory, 2000). Further, Fitzpatrick & LaGory ( 2000) added that these components present at a place shape the lifestyle of the people. Place is a critical social factor that plays an important role in the development of lifestyle related diseases. Rural or urban background helps us to know about the effect of locale of living i.e. rural or urban on the health of an individual.

**Table 3.4 Distribution of Healthy/Unhealthy Respondents on the Basis of**

**Rural-Urban Domicile**

| Respondents' Domicile | Health Status | | Total |
|---|---|---|---|
| | Healthy | Unhealthy | |
| Rural | 44 (61.11%) | 28 (38.89%) | 72 (30.00%) |
| Urban | 66 (39.28%) | 102 (60.71%) | 168 (70.00%) |
| Total | 110 (45.83%) | 130 (54.17%) | 240 (100%) |

Data in Table 3.4 highlight that out of 240 respondents, 72 (30%) belonged to rural areas while 168 (70%) belonged to urban areas. It shows that higher number of urban respondents i.e. 102 (60.71%) were unhealthy as compared to rural respondents i.e. 28

(38.89%). In rural area, there was higher percentage of healthy respondents (61.11%) as compared to unhealthy ones (38.89%). This indicates that rural people may be healthier as compared to the people in urban areas, however we still can see that around 28 (38.89%) of respondents in rural areas had lifestyle related diseases, Therefore, we can witness the penetration of these diseases in rural areas also that illustrates lifestyle related diseases are no longer an 'urban phenomenon'.

**Marital Status**

Marriage may be valuable to health because several spouses observe and try to control the health behaviors of their spouse (Umberson, 1992). Further, Nilsson, Nilson, Ostergren & Berglund (2005) added that there is decreased threat of early death among married, remarried, or cohabiting persons in comparison to those who remain unmarried or are divorced. So, marital status may have an effect on the health of an individual.

Distribution of healthy and unhealthy respondents on the basis of marital status i.e. married, unmarried, divorcee or widow/widower can help us to identify the marital status that is the most and the least affected by the lifestyle related diseases.

**Table 3.5 Distribution of Healthy/Unhealthy Respondents on the
Basis of Marital Status**

| Marital status | Health Status | | Total |
|---|---|---|---|
| | **Healthy** | **Unhealthy** | |
| Married | 97 (48.98%) | 101 ( 51.01%) | 198 (82.92%) |
| Unmarried | 11 (31.42%) | 24 (68.57%) | 35 (14.58%) |
| Widow/Widower | 1 (25.00%) | 3 (75.00%) | 4 (1.67%) |
| Divorcee | 1 (33.33%) | 2 (66.67%) | 3 (1.25%) |
| Total | 110 (45.83%) | 130 (54.17%) | 240 (100%) |

Table 3.5 shows that out of total 240 respondents, 198 (82.92%) were married, 35 (14.58%) were unmarried and 4 (1.67%) were widowers or widows and 3 (1.25%) were divorced. It shows that majority (82.92%) of the respondents were married.

The above data indicate that there is a presence of unhealthy respondents in all the categories. However, the percentage of unhealthy respondents was  much higher in case of divorcees (66.67%), unmarried (68.57%) and widowers (75%) as compared to the healthy respondents in these respective categories

This can be attributed to loneliness and lack of support system among single respondents.

Social support system helps in physical and mental wellbeing of a person. This was evident in Case Studies  015 and 016 where due to lack of social and emotional support doctors suffered from lifestyle related diseases.

**Type of Family Structure**

Humans are naturally social, requiring contact with others (Eibl-Eibesfeldt, 1989). Social interaction between the individual and group is considered to be essential for the health of not only a person but also for the social system.

Umberson and Montez (2010) observed that quality and quatitiy of social relationships influence the physical and mental health as well as the health behaviour and mortality risk among people.

Joint family system has many members that may result in to an increased social interaction and community network. Joint family system may act as a social support system for an individual and may have a positive effect on the physical and psychological health of an individual. Whereas nuclear family structure consists of husband, wife and unmarried children and due to its small size, social interaction  and social support system may be less as compared to joint family structure. Thus it was decided to know about the type of family structure of healthy and unhealthy respondents.

**Table 3.6 Distribution of Healthy/Unhealthy Respondents on the Basis of Family Structure**

| Family Type | Health Status | | Total |
|---|---|---|---|
| | **Healthy** | **Unhealthy** | |
| Nuclear | 50 (37.88%) | 82 (62.12%) | 132 (55.00%) |
| Joint | 60 (55.56%) | 48 (44.44%) | 108 (45.00%) |
| Total | 110 (41.67%) | 130 (54.17%) | 240 (100%) |

Table 3.6 depicts that out of total of 108 (45%) joint families, number of healthy respondents i.e. 60 (55.56%) was higher whereas out of 132 (55%) nuclear families, number of unhealthy respondents was higher i.e. 82 (62.12%).

The data indicate joint family system as a social support system may be conducive to overall health of a person because more number of healthy respondents i.e. 60 (55.56%) healthy as compared to unhealthy i.e. 48 (44.44%) were found in joint family system. There were 82 (62.12%) unhealthy respondents as compared to 50 (37.88%) healthy respondents in nuclear family structure.

**Income per Annum**

Income per annum reflects the socio-economic status of an individual. It is generally believed that higher income brings with it a number of luxuries like motorized vehicles, A.C, electric gadgets etc. at home and work place. Modern facilities further provide impetus to luxurious and sedentary lifestyle and hence, more likelihood of development of lifestyle related diseases. Moreover, while discussing the effect of change in economic condition on the health, Ruhm (2000) found a positive relationship between improvement in financial condition and an increase in risk factors like physical inactivity, obesity and smoking and unhealthy diet.

Income per annum in case of healthy and unhealthy respondents tell us that to which income group the maximum or minimum number of healthy and unhealthy respondents were related. In this way, effect of the income on the health of an individual can be recognized.

**Table 3.7 Distribution of Healthy/Unhealthy Respondents on the Basis of**

**Income per Annum (in Lacs)**

| Income per Annum | Health Status | | Total |
|---|---|---|---|
| | **Healthy** | **Unhealthy** | |
| <10 lacs | 37 (55.22%) | 30 (44.78%) | 67 (27.91%) |
| 10-20 lacs | 40 (41.67%) | 56 (58.33%) | 96 (40.00%) |
| >20 lacs | 33 (42.86%) | 44 (57.14%) | 77 (32.08%) |
| Total | 110 (45.83%) | 130 (54.17%) | 240 (100%) |

As shown in the Table 3.7, there were 40 (41.67%) healthy and 56 (58.33%) unhealthy respondents earning within the range of 10-20 lacs per annum. There were 37 (55.22%) healthy respondents and 30 (44.78%) unhealthy respondents in the income group of <10 lacs per annum, and 33 (42.86%) healthy and 44 (57.14%) unhealthy respondents were in the income group of >20 lacs.

Thus in the relatively higher income group i.e. 10-20 lacs and above 20 lacs per annum, number of unhealthy respondents (58.33% and 57.14% respectively) was more than number of healthy respondents (41.67% and 42.86% respectively) in the same income groups. While in the income group of < 10 lacs the number of healthy respondents (55.22%) was more than the number of unhealthy respondents (44.78%).

The data indicate that as the income level increases, the possibility of unhealthy, materialistic and sedentary lifestyle may increase that can be the possible reason for occurrence of lifestyle related diseases.

**II**

## PROFESSIONAL PROFILE OF RESPONDENTS

Professional profile of healthy and unhealthy respondents has been compared on the basis of area of specialization, type of working institution, nature of job, number of working hours per day, number of working days per week etc. to find out the effect of these factors on the health of the respondents.

### Area of Specialization

Area of specialization depicts the specialization in different branches of medical stream. As mentioned earlier, some medical branches i.e. clinical branches are regarded as to have more stressful working conditions than the non-clinical branches. For instance, Surgery, Gynecology, Orthopedics etc. are believed to be more stressful than Anatomy, Pathology etc. The number of unhealthy and healthy respondents in different areas of specialization will tell about the effect of area of specialization on the health of doctors.

**Table 3.8 (a) Distribution of Healthy/Unhealthy Respondents on the Basis of Area of Specialization (Non-clinical Branches)**

| Non-clinical Branches | Health Status | | Total |
|---|---|---|---|
| | Healthy | Unhealthy | |
| Anatomy | 6 (54.54%) | 5 (45.45%) | 11(15.06%) |
| Physiology | 5 (71.42%) | 2 (28.57%) | 7 (9.58%) |
| Pharmacology | 5 (31.25%) | 11 (68.75%) | 16 (21.91%) |
| SPM* | 4 (50.00%) | 4 (50.00%) | 8 (10.95%) |
| Pathology | 8 (53.33%) | 7 (46.67%) | 15 (20.54%) |
| Microbiology | 1 (20.00%) | 4 (80.00%) | 5 (6.84%) |
| Forensic | 4 (66.67%) | 2 (33.33%) | 6 (8.21%) |
| Biochemistry | 3 (60.00%) | 2 (40.00%) | 5 (6.84%) |
| Total | 36 (49.31%) | 37 (50.68%) | 73 (100%) |

*SPM- Social and Preventive Medicine

Data in the Table 3.8 (a) specify that there were 73 respondents from non-clinical branches i.e. Anatomy, Physiology, Pharmacology, Bio-chemistry etc. of medical field. Among these 73 respondetns, 36 (49.31%) were healthy and 37 (50.68%) were unhealthy.

**Table 3.8 (b) Distribution of Healthy/Unhealthy Respondents on the Basis of Area of Specialization (Clinical Branches)**

| Clincal Branches | Health Status | | Total |
|---|---|---|---|
| | Healthy | Unhealthy | |
| Surgery | 8 (29.62%) | 19 (70.37%) | 27 (16.16%) |
| Skin | 2 (33.33%) | 4 (66.67%) | 6 (3.59%) |
| Ortho | 8 (50.00%) | 8 (50.00%) | 16 (9.58%) |
| Medicine | 23 (46.00%) | 27 (54.00%) | 50 (29.94%) |
| Pediatrics | 2 (50.00%) | 2 (50.00%) | 4 (2.39%) |
| Gynecology | 13 (46.42%) | 15 (53.57%) | 28 (16.76%) |
| Eye | 6 (54.54%) | 5 (45.45%) | 11 (6.58%) |
| ENT* | 6 (75.00%) | 2 (25.00%) | 8 (4.79%) |
| Psychiatry | 2 (25.00%) | 6 (75.00%) | 8 (4.79%) |
| Radiotherapy | 3 (75.00%) | 1 (25.00%) | 4 (2.39%) |
| Anesthesia | 1 (20.00%) | 4 (80.00%) | 5 (2.99%) |
| Total | 74 (44.32%) | 93 (55.68%) | 167 (100%) |

*ENT- Ear, Nose and Trachea

Table 3.8 (b) shows distribution of healthy and unhealthy respondents on the basis of clinical branches i.e. Surgery, Eye, ENT, Pediatrics, Gynecology etc. of medical system. Out of total 167 respondents from clinical branches, 74 (44.33%) were healthy and 93 (55.68%) were unhealthy.

Hence, Table 3.8 (a) specifies that there was almost equal number of healthy (49.31%) and unhealthy (50.68%) respondents in case of non-clinical branches whereas Table 3.8 (b) indicates that number of unhealthy respondents (55.68%) was more than healthy respondents (44.32%) in case of clinical branches. This may be due to busy and irregular work schedule in certain area of specialization i.e. clinical branches that may lead to unhealthy lifestyle and ultimately causation of lifestyle related diseases.

**Type of Working Institution**

Type of working institution i.e. private and public has different kind of work culture. Working environment may have effect on the health of an individual. So, it was an area of interest for the researcher to see whether the type of working institution has any effect on the health of an individual or not. This can be seen by differentiating the number of healthy and unhealthy respondents working in these institutions.

**Table 3.9 Distribution of Healthy/Unhealthy Respondents on the Basis of Type of Working Institution**

| Institution Type | Health Status | | Total |
| --- | --- | --- | --- |
| | Healthy | Unhealthy | |
| Private | 24 (35.82%) | 43 (64.18%) | 67 (27.91%) |
| Public | 86 (49.71%) | 87 (50.29%) | 173 (72.08%) |
| Total | 110 (45.83%) | 130 (54.17%) | 240 (100%) |

The above Table 3.9 depicts that out of 67 (27.91%) respondents working in private institutions, 24 (35.82%) respondents were healthy and 43 (64.18%) were unhealthy whereas among those working in public institutions, number of healthy and unhealthy respondents was 86 (49.71%) and 87 (50.29%) respectively.

The data indicate that government institutions as compared to private institutions had more number of healthy respondents whereas there was higher percentage of unhealthy respondents (64.18%) in private institutions as compared to unhealthy respondents (50.29%) in public institutions. This may be owing to the fixed emoluments as well as working hours in government hospitals whereas lack of job security and uncertain working hours at work place may be the reason for higher number of unhealthy respondents in private hospitals.

In Focused Group Discussion, Dr. B who is working in a private hospital talked about stress in private institutions due to lack of job security and long working hours. Also, many of the doctors were of the view that working in government institutions is relatively less stressful.

**Nature of Job**

As explained in previous chapter there are four main working domains of medical profession viz. OPD (Outdoor Patients), IPD (Indoor patients), both OPD and IPD and Teaching in medical college. They may differ in the work culture and work pressure.

Working in OPD and teaching is assumed to be relaxed, less stressful and less hectic as compared to working in IPD and both OPD and IPD. So, we want to identify the effect of different working domains on health of respondents.

**Table 3.10 Distribution of Healthy/Unhealthy Respondents on the Basis of Nature of Job**

| Nature of Job | Health Status | | Total |
|---|---|---|---|
| | Healthy | Unhealthy | |
| OPD* | 25 (52.08%) | 23 (47.91%) | 48 (20.00%) |
| IPD** | 2 (40.00%) | 3 (60.00%) | 5 (2.08%) |
| Both (OPD & IPD) | 61 (41.78%) | 85 (58.21%) | 146 (60.83%) |
| Teaching | 22 (53.66%) | 19 (46.34%) | 41 (17.08%) |
| Total | 110 (45.83%) | 130 (54.17%) | 240 (100%) |

*OPD-Out door Patient    **IPD-In door Patient

Data in the above Table 3.10 depict that out of total 146 (60.83%) respondents working both in OPD & IPD, 85 (58.21%) were unhealthy and 61 (41.78%) were healthy. In case of respondents working in OPD, 23 (47.91%) were unhealthy and 25 (52.08%) were healthy. Out of 41 (17.08%) respondents working in teaching, 19 (46.34%) were unhealthy and 22 (53.66%) were healthy and there were 3 (60%) unhealthy and 2 (40%) healthy respondents working in IPD.

Thus, data indicate that percentage of unhealthy respondents was more in IPD (60%) and in both OPD and IPD (58.21%) as compared to healthy respondents in these respective categories (40% and 41.78% respectively) and percentage of healthy respondents was more in OPD (52.08%) and teaching domain (53.66%) as compared to unhealthy respondents in the same domains (47.91% and 46.34% respectively)

In case of OPD and teaching, percentage of unhealthy respondents was less. This may be attributable to the lower stress level and fixed duty hours involved in case of teaching and OPD  whereas percentage of unhealthy respondents in IPD and in both OPD and IPD was higher than that of healthy respondents in these respective domains.The reason may be hectic and stressful work schedule in IPD and in both OPD and IPD.

During the Focused Group Discussion, one of the participants Dr. B also discussed his hectic work schedule because he has to manage both OPD and IPD wings of the hospital.

**Experience of Medical Practice**

Duration of practice/job tells about the number of years an individual put in to the practice or job. It also helps us to make out the effect of duration of practice/job on the health of respondent. Question was asked related to the time span of practice or job.

**Table 3.11 Distribution of Healthy/Unhealthy Respondents on the Basis of**

**Years of Medical Practice**

| Years of Medical Practice | Health Status | | Total |
|---|---|---|---|
| | Healthy | Unhealthy | |
| 0-10 | 30 (62.50%) | 18 (37.50%) | 48 (20.00%) |
| 11-20 | 41 (59.42%) | 28 (40.58%) | 69 (28.75%) |
| 21-30 | 29 (45.31%) | 35 (54.69%) | 64 (26.67%) |
| 31-40 | 4 (9.76%) | 37 (90.24%) | 41 (17.08%) |
| 41-50 | 6 (40.00%) | 9 (60.00%) | 15 (6.25%) |
| Above 50 | 0 (0.00%) | 3 (100%) | 3 (1.25%) |
| Total | 110 (45.83%) | 130 (54.17%) | 240 (100%) |

As shown in the above Table 3.11, number of healthy respondents were 41 (59.42%) in 11-20 years of practice, 30 (62.50%) in 0-10 years of practice and 29 (45.31%) in 21-30 years of practice. Other 6 (40%) healthy respondents were in 41-50 years of practice, 4 (9.76%) in 31-40 years of practice and there was no healthy respondent practicing for more than 50 years.

In case of unhealthy respondents, 37 (90.24%) were in 31-40 years of practice, 35 (54.69%) were 21-30 years of practice and 28 (40.58%) were in 11-20 years of practice. Further, 18 (37.50%) were in 0-10 years of practice, 9 (60%) respondents were in 41-50 years of practice and all the 3 (100%) unhealthy respondents in above 50 years of practice.

This data indicate that up to the duration of 20 years of practice/job, number of healthy respondents i.e. 71 was more than the number of unhealthy respondents i.e. 46 but for 21-30 years of practice/job, number of unhealthy respondents (35) outnumbered healthy respondents (29). For 31-40 years of practice/job the difference in number between healthy and unhealthy respondents widened. The number of unhealthy respondents rose to approximately ten times (37) as compared to healthy respondents (4) when duration of practice reached 31-40 years.

Thus as the duration of practice increased i.e. after 20 years of practice the number of unhealthy respondents was more as compared to healthy ones. The maximum number of healthy respondents i.e. 41 out of 110 was found in 11-20 years of practice and maximum number of unhealthy respondents i.e. 37 out of 130 was seen in 31-40 years of duration of work. This indicates that those with long years of practice have more chances of being unhealthy.

**Number of Working Days per Week**

As already said, the number of working days may also affect the health of an individual. To know actually the effect of working days per week on the respondents, the researcher tried to find out the number of healthy and unhealthy respondents working 7 days and less than 7 days a week.

**Table 3.12 Distribution of Healthy/Unhealthy Respondents on the Basis of**

**Number of Working Days per Week**

| Working Days per Week | Health Status | | Total |
|---|---|---|---|
| | **Healthy** | **Unhealthy** | |
| 7 days | 35 (37.63%) | 58 (62.36%) | 93 (38.75%) |
| < 7 days | 75 (51.10%) | 72 (48.97%) | 147 (61.25%) |
| Total | 110 (45.83%) | 130 (54.17%) | 240 (100%) |

The Table 3.12 depicts that out of total 93 (38.75%) respondents working for the whole week without a break, higher number i.e. 58 (62.36%) were unhealthy. The percentage difference between healthy and unhealthy for this category is about 25%.

Out of 147 (61.25%), taking break at least once in a week, 75 (51.10%) were healthy and 72 (48.97%) were unhealthy. Larger numbers of respondents (51.10%) in this category were in healthy state. So, the data indicates that continuous work without any break has a potential of creating a harmful effect on the health of respondents.

In Case Studies 003 (suffering from hypertension) and 009 (suffering from cardiac problem), doctors told that they worked seven days a week without any break whereas Case 013, living a healthy life, enjoys working seven days a week.

**Number of Duty Hours per Day**

The number of working hours per day also reflects the work pressure and daily schedule of the respondents. Working hours beyond a certain limit may not only affect the efficiency of work but also possibly have a bad outcome for the health of an individual. Working for more hours has a negative effect on the lifestyle and daily life of people. The people with lengthy work schedule may not only more liable to smoking, less involved in physical activity and poor sleep but also had poor dietary habits and reduced health examination (Maruyama et al., 1995).

To identify the effect of number of working hours on the health of respondents, question was asked from respondents about the duration of work schedule per day.

**Table 3.13 Distribution of Healthy/Unhealthy Respondents on the Basis of Number of Duty Hours per Day**

| Daily Working Hours | Health Status | | Total |
|---|---|---|---|
| | Healthy | Unhealthy | |
| > 8 hours | 33 (41.77%) | 46 (58.23%) | 79 (32.91%) |
| < 8 hours | 38 (50.67%) | 37 (49.33%) | 75 (31.25%) |
| Depends upon the situation | 39 (45.35%) | 47 (54.65%) | 86 (35.83%) |
| Total | 110 (45.83%) | 130 (54.17%) | 240 (100%) |

Data in the Table 3.13 specifies that out of total 79 (32.91%) respondents working more than 8 hours a day, most of them i.e. 46 ( 58.23%) were unhealthy as compared to 33 (41.77%) healthy respondents. Out of total 75 (31.25%) respondents working less than 8 hours a day, 38 (50.67%) were healthy and 37 (49.33%) were unhealthy. For those who didn't have any fix schedule and their work schedule depends upon the situation were mostly (54.65%) unhealthy. So, number of duty hours shows an effect on the health of respondents.

In Case Studies e.g. Case no. 003 is working more than 8 hours a day. Case no. 009 mentioned that his working hours depended upon the situation. Importantly, doctors in both the cases are unhealthy. On the other hand Case no. 013 despite working for more than 8 hours a day is not stressed at all and leading a healthy life.

Therefore, it can be summed up from the data that continuous and long working hours are found to have negative effect on the health of physicians. The findings in this case corroborate the results of studies  that have found the adverse effect of continuous and long working hours on the cognitive and clinical performance (Philibert, 2005) and diagnostic errors, occupational injuries, motor vehicle accidents etc. (Lockley et al., 2007) among healthcare providers.

**SUMMARY**

A comparison was made between the healthy and unhealthy respondents on the basis of their socio-demographic, economic and professional profiles. As the age of an individual increased, there were more incidences of development of lifestyle related diseases as compared to those who were young in age. Maximum number (52.56%) of healthy respondents falls in age group of 41-50 years whereas maximum number (60.29%) of unhealthy respondents was in age group of 51-60 years. As the age advances beyond 50 years, the percentage of unhealthy respondents increased in comparison to healthy ones.

As per the data of the respondents,  men (59.31%) were more in danger of suffering from these diseases as compared to women (46.31%). All communities like Hindu (57.25%), Sikh (52.53%), Christian, (33.33%) and Muslims (28.57%) were affected by lifestyle related diseases. There were higher incidences of lifestyle related diseases among urban respondents (60.71%) as compared to respondents in rural areas (38.89%).

Further, social support system and close family ties also found to be favorable for the overall well-being of the respondents. There was more number of unhealthy respondents in single marital status such as unmarried (68.57%), widow (75%) or divorcee (66.67%) as compared to married respondents (51.01%). Also, number of unhealthy respondents living in nuclear family structure (62.12%) was more in comparison to those living in joint family structure (44.44%).

As far as the economic profile of healthy and unhealthy respondents was concerned, increased income level also had negative effect on the health of an individual. The number of unhealthy respondents was high in income group 10-20 lacs (58.33%) and >20 lacs (57.14%) per annum as compared to unhealthy respondents in income group less than 10 lacs (44.78%) per annum.

While comparing the professional profiles of healthy and unhealthy respondents, it was found that there was higher number of unhealthy respondents in clinical branches (71.53%) in comparison to non-clinical branches (28.46%) of medical System. The reason may be that work schedule in clinical branches was more hectic as compared to non-clinical branches. The percentage of unhealthy respondents (64.18%)  was more in private institutions as compared to those working in government institutions (50.29%).

Number of years put in to practice or job may also affect the health of the respondents. A continuous increase in the number of unhealthy respondents in comparison to healthy ones was observed after 20 years of practice. The number of unhealthy respondents was more in IPD (60%) and both OPD and IPD (58.21%) in comparison to that of healthy respondents  in IPD (40%) and both OPD and IPD (41.78%) whereas healthy respondents were more in number in OPD (52.08%) and teaching domain (53.66%) in contrast to those of unhealthy respondents working in OPD (47.91%) and teaching (46.34%).  This shows the nature of job affects the health of the individuals.

Further, effect of working hours per day and working days per week has also been observed in the study. The unhealthy respondents working seven days a week without a break and more than eight hours a day were higher in number  (62.36% and 58.23% respectively) as compared to unhealthy respondents working less than seven days a week and less than eight hours a day (48.97% and  49.33% respectively). Hence, in this chapter socio-demographic, economic and professional profile of healthy and unhealthy respondents was discussed so as to be familiar with the effect of profiles on the health of the respondents.

# CHAPTER IV

## LIFESTYLE AND RISK FACTORS: A COMPARISON BETWEEN HEALTHY AND UNHEALTHY RESPONDENTS

Lifestyle of a person can be measured as the sum total of habits, behavior, attitudes etc. that affect the daily life of an individual. These impacts are visible in day to day activities. The physical well-being of an individual can be promoted if behaviors like healthy diet, regular physical workout, adequate sleep and non-consumption of tobacco and alcohol etc. are followed properly. However, if these healthy habits are ignored, they manifest as risk factors responsible for the onset of lifestyle related diseases.

According to WHO and FAO (2003), development of lifestyle related diseases in both developed and developing countries are due to changes in diet and lifestyle. There is a rapid change in the diet and lifestyle of the people due to process of urbanization, industrialization, globalization, and economic development etc. Food and food products, once considered as the basic necessity of life, are now commercialized. The change in food economy all over world resulted in a major shift in dietary pattern that is mainly consisting of saturated fat and refined carbohydrates. This has led to a great impact on the health and nutritional status of people in the developing countries.

Moreover, motorized transport, excessive use of machines at home and work place resulted in to low physical activity. Leisure time activities e.g. watching television, using internet etc. nowadays have become more and more indoor and sedentary in nature. This sedentary lifestyle and changed dietary pattern resulted in to an increase in obesity, heart diseases, diabetes, hypertension, stroke and some types of cancer.

Further, Ziglio, Currie & Rasmussen (2004) mentioned, "WHO stated that 60% of factors related to individual health and quality of life are correlated to lifestyle". Also, various studies indicate that the unhealthy lifestyle of individuals plays an important role in the development of diseases. For instance, Willet et al. (2006) discussed that most of the incidences of heart diseases, diabetes, cancers and stroke can be prevented by reducing recognized modifiable dietary as well as lifestyle risk factors.

WHO (1999) has enlisted diabetes, cardiac problem, asthma and cancer as common lifestyle related diseases and recognized a number of risk factors related to lifestyle and daily habits of the people that are responsible for the development of these diseases (WHO, 2005). These risk factors are i) unhealthy diet, ii) lack of physical exercise iii) tobacco consumption iv) excessive use of alcohol v) obesity vi) high blood pressure vii) high cholesterol level etc. Among these risk factors, unhealthy diet, physical inactivity, excessive use of alcohol and tobacco consumption are called the behaviour risk factors whereas obesity, high blood pressure and high cholesterol level are intermediate risk factors.

In the present study, the researcher was interested in knowing the daily habits such as diet pattern, physical activity, sleeping habits etc. that may affect the lifestyle of both healthy and unhealthy respondents. Therefore, data was collected and analyzed to know about the lifestyle and the prevalence of risk factors among the healthy and unhealthy respondents.

Here, the researcher came across many healthy respondents who were at the risk of developing the lifestyle related diseases because of non-observance of a healthy lifestyle. Besides, there were many unhealthy respondents who preferred to follow a healthy lifestyle after suffering from the diseases. Hence, comparison between healthy and unhealthy respondents can provide key insights into the causation of the lifestyle related diseases among the respondents.

**PERCEPTION ABOUT THEIR LIFESTYLE**

Perception of respondents about lifestyle means type of life the respondents feel or perceive they are living. The lifestyle may be sedentary, moderately active or very much active. According to WHO (2002), a sedentary lifestyle is one of the major risk factors for poor health and reduced functional capability. It is characterized by low physical activity that results in to increase in body weight or obesity. Further, Warburton, Nicol & Bredin (2006) added that sedentary job results in to fewer chances of physical mobility and exercise. This low physical mobility enhances the risk for obesity and chronic diseases like cardiac problems and diabetes (Warburton et al., 2006).

So to be familiar with the lifestyle of the respondents was very important in our study in order to make out the effect of lifestyle on health status of an individual. Question was asked about the perception of respondents about their lifestyles and the comparison was done between the lifestyle of healthy and unhealthy respondents.

**Table 4.1 Distribution of Healthy/Unhealthy Respondents on the Basis of**

**Perception about their Lifestyle**

| Lifestyle | Health Status | | Total |
|---|---|---|---|
| | **Healthy** | **Unhealthy** | |
| Sedentary | 20 (37.74%) | 33 (62.26%) | 53 (22.08%) |
| Moderately active | 60 (40.00%) | 90 (60.00%) | 150 (62.50%) |
| Very much active | 30 (81.08%) | 7 (18.92%) | 37 (15.41%) |
| Total | 110 (45.83%) | 130 (54.17%) | 240 (100%) |

Data in the Table 4.1 show that 150 (62.50%) respondents had 'moderately active' lifestyle. Out of these 150 'moderately active' respondents, 60 (40%) were healthy and 90 (60%) were unhealthy. Out of 53 (22.08%) respondents who had sedentary lifestyle, 20 (37.74%) were healthy and 33 (62.26%) were unhealthy, 37 (15.41%) respondents believed that they had 'very much active' lifestyle and out of these 37 respondents, 30 (81.08%) were healthy and 7 (18.92%) were unhealthy.

Thus, lifestyle of most of the respondents, (about 78% ie moderately and very much active) was more or less active. However, there was small number of respondents (22%) who had sedentary lifestyle. 'Sedentary' lifestyle was more frequent among unhealthy respondents (62.26%) as compared to healthy respondents (37.74%). Among the 'moderately active' respondents, number of unhealthy respondents (60%) was more than healthy respondents (40%), it seems that unhealthy respondents tried to follow a healthy lifestyle by being 'moderately active'. Among the 'very much active' respondents, number of healthy respondents was more than four times i.e. 30 (81.08%) as compared to unhealthy respondents i.e. 7 (18.92%). This indicates that 'very much active' lifestyle helps in keeping oneself healthy.

The above data show that unhealthy respondents with sedentary lifestyle were comparatively higher in number. Further, in Case Studies 002, 007, 008 and 015 it was found that the doctors had sedentary lifestyle and were having different kind of health related problems whereas in Case Study 012, doctor told that he is healthy at the age of 56 years due to his 'very much active' lifestyle.

Similar relation between health and sedentary lifestyle was confirmed in a study by Jardim et al. (2015) that revealed the presence of sedentary lifestyle as one of the risk factors responsible for heart diseases. This indicates that active lifestyle is good for the health of an individual.

## RISK FACTORS

Health and well-being of people may be affected by a number of lifestyle related factors. These factors when manifest in to disease, poor health and disability are known as risk factors. WHO (2005) defined risk factor as "A risk factor refers to any attribute, characteristic, or exposure of an individual, which increases the likelihood of developing a non-communicable disease." Risk factors responsible for chronic diseases, generally, do not occur individually. They are accompanied by some other risk factors. For example, an increase in body weight, blood pressure as well as cholesterol level caused by physical inactivity, finally, results in chronic heart diseases.

Questions were asked from the healthy and unhealthy respondents about the diet, physical activity, consumption of alcohol and tobacco products, sleeping habits etc. to know about the lifestyle and presence of risk factors among respondents.

### Diet

Diet is concerned with the eating habits of an individual. Diet comprises of not only various types of food intake but also quantity and frequency with which they are consumed in routine.

Diet has both positive and negative effects on the health of an individual throughout the lifetime. Dietary pattern not only affects the health of an individual presently but also it is an important determinant whether or not a person will suffer from heart disease, cancer or diabetes in future. Diet is considered as the major modifiable factor for causation of lifestyle related diseases. So, the questions were asked from the respondents about meal schedule i.e. regular or irregular, intake of fruits, vegetables or legumes etc.

*Type of Meal Schedule*

Food and nutrition is the basic necessity of the human beings for the survival as well as for the good health. Regular meal schedule that corresponds to timely intake of three meals in a day is responsible for good health of an individual. Irregular meal schedule involving skipping and ill-timed intake of food results in to obesity, high blood pressure, diabetes, heart disease etc. (St-Onge et al., 2017).

So, it is imperative to know about the meal schedule of the healthy and unhealthy respondents to assess the prevalence of risk factors among respondents.

**Table 4.2 Distribution of Healthy/Unhealthy Respondents on the Basis of**

**Type of Meal Schedule***

| Meal Schedule | Health Status | | Total |
|---|---|---|---|
| | **Healthy** | **Unhealthy** | |
| Regular | 95 (52.19%) | 87 (47.80%) | 182 (75.83%) |
| Irregular | 15 (25.86%) | 43 (74.13%) | 58 (24.16%) |
| Total | 110 (45.83%) | 130 (54.17%) | 240 (100%) |

*3 Meals/day

Table 4.2 indicates that there were 182 (75.83%) respondents who followed a regular meal schedule. Out of these 182 (75.83%) respondents, 95 (52.19%) were healthy and 87 (47.80%) were unhealthy whereas 58 (24.16%) respondents had irregular meal schedule. Out of these 58 respondents, 15 (25.86%) were healthy and 43 (74.13%) were unhealthy.

This shows that maximum number of respondents i.e. 182 had regular meal schedule whereas respondents with irregular meal schedule were small in number i.e. 58.

Also, there was larger number of unhealthy respondents (74.13%) having irregular meal schedule as compared to healthy ones (25.86%). This indicates that irregular meal schedule may act as a risk factor for onset of lifestyle related diseases.

However, there was not much difference in number between the healthy (95) and unhealthy (87) respondents taking regular meal schedule. It seems unhealthy respondents may have started regular meal schedule after the onset of disease.

A number of Cases, for instance, 002, 003,005, 009, 010 mentioned the habit of irregular eating schedule among doctors. In the Focused Group Discussion, most of the participants said that they were irregular in their meal intake because of their hectic work schedule. Thus, irregular meal schedule is not uncommon among doctors who are assumed to be conscious about their dietary intake and health needs.

*Reasons for Irregularity in Meal Schedule*

As said earlier that irregular meal schedule means when respondent is not consuming timely and required frequency of food in a day. Out of total 240 respondents, 58 (24.16%) respondents were having an irregular meal schedule. So, next question was about the reasons for irregularity in food intake among these 58 respondents. There were a number of reasons given for the irregular intake of food by these respondents which are shown in the following table.

**Table 4.3 Distribution of the Respondents on the Basis of Reasons for**

**Irregularity in Meal Schedule**

| Reasons for Irregularity* | Number of Respondents | Percentage |
|---|---|---|
| Busy schedule | 46/58 | 79.31% |
| Lack of appetite | 4/58 | 6.89% |
| Carelessness | 10/58 | 17.24% |
| Other reasons (age factor, health problem etc.) | 3/58 | 5.17% |

* Multiple responses

Table 4.3 depicts the different reasons for the intake of irregular meal schedule like busy schedule, lack of appetite, carelessness etc. The respondents assigned more than one reason for the irregularity in meal schedule. Busy schedule (79.31%) was the main reason assigned for the irregular meal schedule followed by carelessness (17.24%), lack of appetite (6.89%) and other reasons (5.17%).

Since medical profession is one of the busiest professions so the maximum number of respondents i.e. 46 (79.31%) blamed 'busy schedule' for irregular diet pattern. In Case Studies also various reasons were given for irregular eating schedule, e.g., Case

003 blamed carelessness and Case 005 held busy schedule responsible for irregularity whereas Case 010 gave multiple reasons like busy job, irregular shifts and carelessness for irregular meal schedule.

Most of the respondents during Focused Group Discussion told that the most common reason for their irregular meal schedule was their busy work schedule, for instance, Dr. B mentioned that in case of emergency he has to work day and night. Due to this busy work schedule, timely intake of food becomes difficult.

### *Frequency of Dining Outside*

National Restaurant Association (2012) analyzed the data from 'National Health and Nutrition Examination Survey' (1999-2000) and revealed that the average person takes restaurant prepared food approximately three times in a week and frequency of dining out is continuously increasing thereafter (National Restaurant Association, 2012). Moreover, calories in this food are considerably high as compared to home cooked food and thus dining out turns out to be key risk factor for obesity and thus, for heart diseases (Alkerwi, Crichton & Hébert, 2015).

However, frequency of dining outside in restaurants, hotels etc. also indicate about the respondents' level of awareness about the healthy food intake.

**Table 4.4 Distribution of Healthy/Unhealthy Respondents on the Basis of**

**Frequency of Dining Outside**

| Dining Outside | Health Status | | Total |
|---|---|---|---|
| | **Healthy** | **Unhealthy** | |
| Not at all | 10 (66.67%) | 5 (33.33%) | 15 (6.25%) |
| Occasionally | 49 (42.98%) | 65 (57.01%) | 114 (47.50%) |
| 1-2 days/week | 44 (47.83%) | 48 (52.17%) | 92 (38.33%) |
| 3-4 days/week | 6 (37.50%) | 10 (62.50%) | 16 (6.67%) |
| Almost everyday | 1 (33.33%) | 2 (66.67%) | 3 (1.25%) |
| Total | 110 (45.83%) | 130 (54.17%) | 240 (100%) |

Table 4.4 specifies that maximum number of respondents had more or less habit of dining out. There were only 15 (6.25%) respondents in total 240 who were not taking

food outside. Out of these 15 (6.25%) respondents, 10 (66.67%) were healthy and 5 (33.33%) were unhealthy.

Among those i.e. 114 (47.50%) who 'occasionally' went out for dining, 49 (42.98%) were healthy and 65 (57.01%) were unhealthy. Those i.e. 92 (38.33%) respondents who dined outside '1-2 days' in a week, 44 (47.83%) were healthy and 48 (52.17%) were unhealthy. Among 16 (6.67%) respondents who consumed food outside '3-4 days' per week, number of unhealthy respondents (62.50%) was more than healthy respondents (37.50%). The number of unhealthy respondents (66.67%) was double as compared to healthy respondents (33.33%) who had the habit of dining outside 'almost every day'.

The results showed that both healthy and unhealthy respondents were evenly in the habit of dining outside but unhealthy respondents who dined outside ('occasionally' or '1-2 days' and '3-4 days a week' or 'almost every day') were more in number in comparison to healthy respondents in these respective categories whereas there was double number (66.67%) of healthy respondents as compared to unhealthy respondents (33.33%) who never dined outside. It seems that dining outside may be one of the risk factors for the occurrence of disease.

Cases 003 and 004 mentioned that they had the habit of taking food in restaurants. It is important to refer here that both the cases were unhealthy. Case 003 was hypertensive at the young age of 24 years and Case 004 was hypertensive and suffering from cardiac problem quite early. Both cited unhealthy diet as one of the key factors responsible for hypertension.

During Focused Group Discussion, the majority of the participants mentioned that they have the inclination to dine out or take ready to eat food when there is any get together. Also, some of the doctors said that they generally go outside for dinner on every weekend.

***Frequency of Intake of Junk Food***

A specific definition of junk food is not given anywhere. According to "Food Safety and Standards Act" (2006), eateries like pizzas, burgers, noodles, chips etc. are categorized as "Propriety or novel" food (as cited in Down to Earth, 2015).

In the era of globalization, consumption of junk food becomes the culture of all the developing and developed societies. The big food companies like KFC, McDonald,

Pizza Huts etc. are penetrating in the food culture of developing societies and are replacing the traditional foods with westernized food items. Junk food is highly processed and easy to cook food. This type of food is rich in high levels of sugar, salt, trans-saturated fat and carbohydrates. High levels of these harmful contents result not only in to obesity but also are responsible for increasing burden of non-communicable diseases (Down to Earth, 2015).

It was desired to be acquainted with the health status of the respondents consuming or not consuming junk food. Both healthy and unhealthy respondents were asked question about the frequency of consuming junk food.

**Table 4.5 Distribution of Healthy/Unhealthy Respondents on the Basis of Frequency of Intake of Junk Food**

| Consumption of Junk Food | Health Status | | Total |
|---|---|---|---|
| | **Healthy** | **Unhealthy** | |
| Not at all | 17 (39.53%) | 26 (60.46%) | 43 (17.91%) |
| Occasionally | 72 (48.98%) | 75 (51.02%) | 147 (61.25%) |
| 1-2 days/week | 20 (44.44%) | 25 (55.56%) | 45 (18.75%) |
| 3-4 days/week | 1 (33.33%) | 2 (66.67%) | 3 (1.25%) |
| Almost everyday | 0 (0.00%) | 2 (100%) | 2 (0.83%) |
| Total | 110 (45.83%) | 130 (54.17%) | 240 (100%) |

As shown in the Table 4.5, most of the respondents (about 82%) were taking junk food. There were only 18% respondents who were not taking junk food. Higher number (60.46%) of unhealthy respondents were found in comparison to healthy ones (39.53%) who were not   consuming junk food. It seems that unhealthy respondents are refraining from taking junk food after the occurrence of diseases.

There was not much difference in number of healthy (72) and unhealthy (75) respondents consuming junk food 'occasionally'. Those consuming junk food '1-2 days' a week, 25 (55.56%) were unhealthy and 20 (44.44%) were healthy. There were 2 (66.67%) unhealthy respondents and 1 (33.33%) healthy respondent eating junk food '3-4 days' a week. Those consuming junk food 'everyday', all were unhealthy i.e. 2 (100%).

In Cases 004 and 008 also, habit of eating junk food frequently has been reported.

Data show that as the frequency of taking junk food increases from 'occasionally' to 'everyday', the percentage of unhealthy respondents rises constantly in comparison to healthy respondents. This indicates that frequent intake of junk food may have negative effect on the health of the respondents.

### *Frequency of Consumption of Milk Products*

Milk and milk products are considered as a major source of protein. Consumption of one serving of milk (250 ml.) and two servings of curd are ideal for the health of an individual (Rayomand Engineer, 2018) whereas two servings of milk and milk products per day are said to be good for the health of an individual.

Doctors are the learned people who are entirely aware about the healthy dietary pattern. So, we wanted to get information about the frequency of intake of milk and milk products from healthy and unhealthy respondents to make out the effect of milk and milk products consumption on the health of respondents.

**Table 4.6 Distribution of Healthy/Unhealthy Respondents on the Basis**

**Frequency of Consumption of Milk Products per Day**

| Consumption of Milk Products per Day | Health Status | | Total |
|---|---|---|---|
| | **Healthy** | **Unhealthy** | |
| 2 or >2 servings | 63 (51.22%) | 60 (48.78%) | 123 (51.25%) |
| < 2 servings | 41 (40.20%) | 61 (59.80%) | 102 (42.50%) |
| Hardly consume any milk product | 6 (40.00%) | 9 (60.00%) | 15 (6.25%) |
| Total | 110 (45.83%) | 130 (54.17%) | 240 (100%) |

Table 4.6 depicts that out of those 123 (51.25%) respondents who took 2 or 'more than 2 servings' of milk products/day, 63 (51.22%) respondents were healthy and 60 (48.78%) were unhealthy. There were 102 (42.50%) respondents [41 (40.20%) healthy and 61 (59.80%) unhealthy] who consumed less than 2 servings/day and there were 15 (6.25%) respondents [6 (40%) healthy and 9 (60%) unhealthy] who hardly consumed any milk product.

This indicates that 123 (51.25%) respondents were taking 2 or 'more than 2 servings' per day which was considered to be good for health. However, there was large number of respondents (48.75%) who hardly consume requisite quantity of milk and milk products. This shows the callousness on the part of doctors to follow a healthy diet pattern.

The data show that the respondents consuming 'less than two servings' of milk and milk products are comparatively unhealthier. This confirms unhealthy diet as one of the risk factors for the causation of diseases among respondents. So, consumption of milk and milk products below required quantity has a harmful effect on the health of individuals. Also, we find in Case 004, an unhealthy one, where milk is hardly consumed daily.

### Frequency of Consumption of Fruits and Vegetables/Legumes

According to WHO (2003), five servings or 400 grams of fruits and vegetables or legumes are necessary in daily diet intake. These five servings are vital for fulfilling requirement for healthy and balanced diet. Consumption of fruits and vegetables or legumes lower than the required quantity acts as risk factor for global burden of non-communicable diseases (WHO, 2002).

Survey by 'Department of Women and Child development' (Government of India, 1998) in India reveals that only 120-140 grams of fruits and vegetables are consumed on daily basis which is not according to the prescribed quantity of 400 grams per person per day by WHO. So, question was asked about the intake of fruits and vegetables or legumes to discern the number of servings consumed by the healthy and unhealthy respondents.

**Table 4.7 Distribution of Healthy/Unhealthy Respondents on the Basis of Frequency of Consumption of Fruits and Vegetables or Legumes per Day**

| Consumption of Fruits and Vegetables or Legumes per Day | Health Status | | Total |
|---|---|---|---|
| | Healthy | Unhealthy | |
| 5 servings or more/day | 9 (42.85%) | 12 (57.14%) | 21 (8.75%) |
| 4 servings /day | 62 (44.28%) | 78 (55.71%) | 140 (58.33%) |
| 3 servings /day | 39 (50.00%) | 39 (50.00%) | 78 (32.50%) |
| 2 servings /day | 0 (0.00%) | 1 (100%) | 1 (0.41%) |
| 1 servings /day | 0 (0.00%) | 0 (0.00%) | 0 (0.00%) |
| No serving | 0 (0.00%) | 0 (0.00%) | 0 (0.00%) |
| Total | 110 (45.83%) | 130 (54.17%) | 240 (100%) |

The data in the Table 4.7 indicate that only 21 (8.75%) respondents met the WHO requirement of number of fruits and vegetables/legumes servings per day. Further, 140 (58.33%) were close to the prescribed requirements. However, rest of nearly 33% did not meet the WHO recommendations of five servings of fruits and vegetables or legumes per day.

Thus, larger number of unhealthy respondents i.e. 90 out of 130 were fulfilling (5 servings or more) or almost fulfilling (4 servings) the guidelines of WHO of taking '5 servings' of fruits and vegetables or legume per day as compared to 71 out of 110 healthy respondents. It appears that unhealthy respondents are trying to follow a healthy lifestyle after falling ill.

The above trend of consumption of fruits and vegetables or legumes shows that there is more inclination of unhealthy respondents towards taking required amount of healthy diet to maintain a good health while healthy respondents showed less inclination towards healthy diet pattern and thus, increasing the risk for lifestyle related diseases.

In Case Studies 003, 004, 008 it was found that low intake of fruits, vegetables or legumes resulted in to onset of one or the other type of lifestyle related disease.

In Focused Group Discussion, all the participants were not aware about the WHO recommendation of healthy and balanced diet in the form of five servings of fruits and vegetables or legumes whereas some other mentioned that they tried to follow the recommendations but could not do this on regular basis.

Therefore, WHO's prescription of five servings of fruits and vegetables or legumes are important for good health of individuals.

**Physical Activity**

WHO (2010) enlisted physical inactivity as the fourth main reason for mortality due to non-communicable or lifestyle related diseases after high blood pressure, overweight and high blood glucose level. It recommends 150 minutes per week for moderate intensity exercise and 75 minutes per week for vigorous intensity exercise spread over whole week.

Physical activity plays an important role in keeping oneself healthy. Lack of physical activity also results in obesity which acts as a risk factor for different types of lifestyle related diseases like heart disease, diabetes, breast cancer etc. Primarily, it is important to look in to the Body Mass Index of the healthy and unhealthy respondents to identify the respondents with overweight.

***Body Mass Index***

According to National Institute of Diabetes, Digestive and Kidney Diseases (NIDDK, 2015), obesity and overweight have many health risks like heart disease, certain cancers, hypertension, osteoarthritis, diabetes etc. In order to maintain a healthy and normal body weight, healthy diet and regular physical exercise is needed.

In the present research, researcher was interested to identify the respondents with healthy and unhealthy range of body weight with the help of Body Mass Index (BMI). BMI (Body Mass Index) is measured by weight in kilogram divided by height in meter$^2$. This may help us to recognize the respondents at risk of developing the above said chronic illnesses associated with overweight.

**Table 4.8 Distribution of Healthy/Unhealthy Respondents on the Basis of**

**BMI (Body Mass Index) in Kg/m$^2$**

| Body Mass Index (Kg/m$^2$) | Health Status | | Total |
|---|---|---|---|
| | Healthy | Unhealthy | |
| Healthy (18.5-24.9) | 64 (56.64%) | 49 (43.36%) | 113 (47.08%) |
| Overweight (25-29.9) | 40 (39.21%) | 62 (60.78%) | 102 (42.50%) |
| Obese (30 and above) | 6 (28.57%) | 15 (71.43%) | 21 (8.75%) |
| Severely obese (>35) | 0 (0.00%) | 4 (100%) | 4 (1.67%) |
| Total | 110 (45.83%) | 130 (54.17%) | 240 (100%) |

Data in the Table 4.8 show that the weight of 64 (56.64%) healthy and 49 (43.36%) unhealthy respondents was in healthy range, 40 (39.21%) healthy and 62 (60.78%) unhealthy respondents were 'overweight', 6 (28.57%) healthy and 15 (71.43%) unhealthy respondents were 'obese', and there was no (0%) healthy and 4 (100%) unhealthy respondents who were 'severely obese' i.e. all the 'severely obese' respondents were unhealthy.

More than half number of respondents i.e. 127 (52.92%) out of 240 fall in unhealthy range of BMI i.e. 'overweight', 'obese' and 'severely obese'. Also, number of unhealthy respondents was more in unhealthy range of BMI as compared to healthy respondents. However, there was higher number of healthy respondents as compared to unhealthy ones within healthy range of BMI.

The above findings indicate that unhealthy respondents with increased body weight was more in number as compared to healthy respondents but incidence of high body weight as risk factor is also visible among healthy respondents.

Moreover, different unhealthy ranges of BMI was found among doctors in many case studies, for instance,  Cases 004 and 007 were overweight, Case 016 was slightly obese, Cases 008, 009 and 015 were obese, and Case 005 was severely obese.

Similar finding is observed by Jardim et al. (2015) among healthcare professionals. The study identified presence of overweight and other risk factors for the causation of heart diseases among medical practitioners.

*Physical Workout*

According to U.S. Department of Health and Human Services (2018), "Being physically active is one of the most important actions that people of all ages can take to improve their health". The subsequent research strengthened this statement and revealed that physical activity may play an important role in lowering risk of high blood pressure, stroke, heart disease, diabetes (Type-2) and some cancers. Physical workout is thus necessary to keep oneself healthy. It helps in keeping the body weight in control. It is desired to check the regularity/irregularity of physical workout to understand the prevalence of this risk factor among healthy and unhealthy respondents.

**Table 4.9 Distribution of Healthy/Unhealthy Respondents on the Basis of Regular Physical Workout**

| Regular Physical    Workout | Health Status | | Total |
|---|---|---|---|
| | **Healthy** | **Unhealthy** | |
| Yes | 72 (52.94%) | 64 (47.06%) | 136 (56.67%) |
| No | 38 (36.53%) | 66 (63.46%) | 104 (43.33%) |
| Total | 110 (45.83%) | 130 (54.17%) | 240 (100%) |

Table 4.9 indicates that 72 (52.94%) healthy and 64 (47.06%) unhealthy respondents were doing regular physical workout whereas 38 (36.53%) healthy and 66 (63.46%) unhealthy were not doing regular physical workout.

The data show that there were good numbers i.e. 104 (43.33%) of respondents who did not have the habit of regular physical workout. However, there were 136 (56.67%) respondents who were regularly doing physical workout.

Moreover, the data show that physical work out has positive effect on the health of respondents. The number of healthy respondents (52.94%) was higher as compared to unhealthy ones (47.06%) who were doing regular physical workout whereas the number of unhealthy respondents (63.46%) was much higher in comparison to healthy respondents (36.53%) who were not doing regular physical workout.

Also, in majority of the Case Studies, low, irregular or absence of physical activity was found among unhealthy doctors, e.g. in 001, 003, 004, 005, 007, 008, 009 Whereas Cases 011, 012, 013 mentioned the habit of regular physical activity and were healthy.

It can be inferred from the above finding that significant number of doctors are not doing physical workout on regular basis. Similar findings about the lack of exercise among doctors were reported by Wada et al. (2011) and Wiskar (2012) in their studies.

*Reasons behind Irregular Physical Activity*

As shown in the above data, a large number of respondents (104 respondents) were not regular in doing physical exercise in their day to day life, so to explore the reasons behind this irregularity, the researcher tried to find out the barriers against physical activity by asking question related to it.

**Table 4.10 Distribution of Respondents' Perception of**

**Barriers Against Physical Activity**

| Barrier Against Physical Activity* | Number of respondents | Percentage |
|---|---|---|
| Busy schedule | 68/104 | 65.38% |
| Lack of interest | 24/104 | 23.07% |
| Health related problem | 24/104 | 23.07% |
| Lack of practical conditions | 19/104 | 18.26% |
| Too tired | 29/104 | 27.88% |
| Callousness | 6/104 | 5.76% |
| No specific reason | 4/104 | 3.84% |

*Multiple Responses

Table 4.10 focuses on the barriers felt by the respondents against the physical activity. Here respondents assigned multiple reasons for not doing the physical workout. Maximum number of respondents i.e. 68 (65.38%) felt their busy schedule as the barrier against physical activity, 29 (27.88%) respondents were too tired to perform physical activity, 24 (23.07%) respondents showed lack of interest, 24 (23.07%) respondents perceived health related problem and 19 (18.26%) respondents blamed lack of practical conditions as barrier against physical activity. Rest 6 (5.76%) respondents told callousness and 4 (3.84%) assigned no specific reason as the barrier against the physical activity.

The maximum number of respondents (68) assigned busy schedule as the barrier against the physical activity because medical profession is considered to be a time and energy demanding profession. Doctors have to work day and night without a fixed time schedule. Such a demanding profession also results in to tiredness that acts as barrier against the physical activity. Moreover, some respondents came up with the reason of lack of practical conditions like winters, pollution or gym at the far off place etc. and some talked about their health related issues like arthritis, asthma etc. as the barrier against physical activity. Some respondents held their callousness and lack of interest responsible for not doing the physical activity.

Case Studies 003 and 016 blamed busy schedule, Case 010 said lack of time and Case 009 mentioned poor health condition along with busy schedule as the reasons for low as well as  lack of physical activity.

During Focused Group Discussion, most of the participants said that they generally do not engage in the physical workout.  They said that most of them are too busy and ambitious for their career growth to have time for physical activity. Few of them said that awful health situation or lack of practical conditions may be the reason for lack of physical activity. One of the participants, Dr. E, blamed his asthmatic problem and another participant, Dr. J, held arthritis responsible for lack of physical activity.

### *Preference for Type of Physical Workout*

As already said, there were 136 respondents doing regular physical workout or activity. Stretching or strengthening, walking, aquatic or swimming and bicycling are the different forms of exercises. Some exercises are known to be as low intensity exercises i.e. walking and some are of moderate or high intensity in nature like swimming and bicycling. Some other exercises are of high intensity exercises like stretching or strengthening exercises or brisk walking etc.  Researcher was interested to know about the type of exercise preferred by the 136 respondents having the habit of regular physical workout.

**Table 4.11 Distribution of Healthy/Unhealthy Respondents on the Basis of**

**Type of Physical Workout Preferred**

| Type of Physical Workout Preferred | Health Status | | Total* |
|---|---|---|---|
| | **Healthy** | **Unhealthy** | |
| Walking | 30 (35.39%) | 55 (64.70%) | 85 (62.50%) |
| Bicycling | 13 (72.22%) | 5 (27.78%) | 18 (13.23%) |
| Swimming | 5 (71.42%) | 2 (28.57%) | 7 (5.14%) |
| Stretching or Strengthening | 41 (73.21%) | 15 (26.78%) | 56 (41.17%) |

*Multiple Responses

Table 4.11 depicts that majority of the respondents i.e. 85 (62.50%) preferred walk as an exercise, 56 (41.17%) respondents were doing stretching or strengthening exercises, bicycling and swimming were preferred by 18 (13.23%) and 7 (5.14%) respondents respectively.

Out of 85 respondents doing walk as an exercise, 55 (64.70%) were unhealthy and 30 (35.39%) were healthy whereas 41 (73.21%) healthy and 15 (26.78%) unhealthy respondents preferred stretching or strengthening as a physical activity. Out of 18 respondents preferring bicycling, 13 (72.22%) were healthy and 5 (27.78%) were unhealthy. There were 5 (71.42%) healthy and 2 (28.57%) unhealthy respondents opting for swimming as a type of physical activity.

Thus, data specify that most preferred kind of physical activity by unhealthy respondents was walking whereas healthy respondents mostly preferred stretching or strengthening exercises. From the data, it appears that unhealthy respondents mostly preferred low intensity exercises whereas healthy respondents show inclination towards moderate or high intensity exercises.

**Tobacco Consumption**

Tobacco and tobacco products are not considered good for the health of an individual. There are two types of tobacco products i.e. smoke and smokeless. In smoke tobacco products cigarette, cigar is included while smokeless products are chewing or sniffing tobacco.

A Report of the Surgeon General stated that smoking is not only the main cause of different types of cancers such as cancer of the lung, liver, kidney, pancreas etc. but also responsible for chronic obstructive pulmonary disease (COPD), heart disease, respiratory disease, diabetes and rheumatoid arthritis (Human and Health Services, 2014). The persons taking these products are at the risk of suffering from lifestyle related diseases.

*Presence/Absence of Tobacco Consumption*

As said previously that consuming tobacco products are harmful for the health of the individuals. So, it was important to discern the habit of tobacco consumption among the respondents. Question related to the presence of the tobacco consumption (now or ever) was asked from respondents to recognize the habit of tobacco consumption among respondents.

**Table 4.12 Distribution of Healthy/Unhealthy Respondents on the Basis of**

**Consumption of Tobacco Products (now or ever)**

| Consumption of Tobacco (now or ever) | Health Status | | Total |
|---|---|---|---|
| | Healthy | Unhealthy | |
| Yes | 22 (37.93%) | 36 (62.07%) | 58 (24.17%) |
| No | 88 (48.35%) | 94 (51.65%) | 182 (75.83%) |
| Total | 110 (45.83%) | 130 (54.17%) | 240 (100%) |

Table 4.12 indicates that among 58 (24.17%) respondents consuming tobacco products, 36 (62.07%) were unhealthy and 22 (37.93%) were healthy whereas for 182 (75.83%) respondents who never consumed any tobacco products, 88 (48.35%) were healthy and 94 (51.65%) were unhealthy.

There were 58 (24.17%) respondents taking tobacco products and most of them (62.07%) were unhealthy. This shows that consumption of tobacco products is one of the risk factors for the development of disease.

The report of Stepwise survey carried by PGI Chandigarh (PGIMER, 2014) found the number of respondents having habit of consuming tobacco in Punjab is less. However it is still doubtful that whether the respondents have given true information regarding tobacco consumption or have concealed the facts about their addiction to tobacco.

This is commonly believed that cigarette smoking may be the one of the possible reasons for the onset of heart disease. In Case Studies 001 and 004, doctors suffered from cardiac problem and in Case 002, hypertension and cardiac problem was reported due to the habit of smoking.

Many participants during Focused Group Discussion were of the view that tobacco consumption is one of the major risk factors for the development of lifestyle related diseases. One of the participants, Dr. L, assigned cigarette smoking as the reason for his heart problem at a very young age.

The above findings show that there were approximately one fourth of the respondents consuming tobacco products. It is relevant to mention here the study by Wada et al. (2011) that observed the smoking habit among physician.

**Alcohol Consumption**

According to WHO (1999), the ideal recommended quantity of pure alcohol intake is about 20-25 gram per day. Further, WHO recommends consumption of two standard units or less than two standard units per day with at least two non-drinking days per week. According to WHO, one standard unit equals to 10g of pure ethanol. It is considered that recommended quantity of alcohol has medicinal value but in excess quantity it is harmful for a person.

So, in our research we tried to know about the frequency of taking alcohol in a week, numbers of drinks taken per day, change in quantity of alcohol over time and duration of consuming alcohol among the healthy and unhealthy respondents. This may help in determining the effect of consuming alcohol on the health of respondents.

*Presence/Absence of Alcohol Consumption*

Presence of habit of alcohol intake plays an important role for the health of an individual. So, researcher wanted to identify the number of respondents consuming alcohol.

**Table 4.13 Distribution of Healthy/Unhealthy Respondents on the Basis of**

**Consumption of Alcohol**

| Consumption of Alcohol | Health Status | | Total |
|---|---|---|---|
| | Healthy | Unhealthy | |
| Yes | 42 (42.00%) | 58 (58.00%) | 100 (41.67%) |
| No | 68 (48.57%) | 72 (51.43%) | 140 (58.33%) |
| Total | 110 (45.83%) | 130 (54.17%) | 240 (100%) |

Table 4.13 specifies that most of respondents i.e. 140 (58.33%) were not taking alcohol and among these respondents, 68 (48.57%) were healthy and 72 (51.43%) were unhealthy. There were 42 (42%) healthy and 58 (58%) unhealthy respondents out of total 100 (41.67%) respondents taking alcohol.

The data show that number of unhealthy respondents (58%) taking alcohol was more than the healthy respondents (42%). There was small difference in number between healthy and unhealthy respondents who were not taking alcohol. This shows that alcohol consumption may negatively affect the health of an individual. Thus alcohol consumption may be one of the risk factors for the causation of disease.

Moreover, habit of alcohol consumption was also found among the doctors in Case Studies 001, 002 and 004. Importantly, all of these cases were found to be unhealthy.

Similar finding is reflected in the study of Jardim et al. (2015) where alcohol consumption was one of the risk factors for the occurrence of heart diseases among physicians.

### Frequency of Abstaining from Alcohol in a Week

Frequency of abstaining from alcohol per week indicates the number of times in a week the respondents refrain from taking alcohol. The WHO (1999) recommends that an individual should abstain from alcohol for at least two days per week for optimum health. So it was asked to the respondents about the approximate number of days of the week when they can avoid alcohol

**Table 4.14 Distribution of Healthy/Unhealthy Respondents on the Basis**

**Frequency of Abstaining from Alcohol Consumption**

| Abstaining from Alcohol Consumption | Health Status | | Total |
|---|---|---|---|
| | Healthy | Unhealthy | |
| Abstaining more than a week | 24 (85.71%) | 4 (14.29%) | 28 (28.00%) |
| Abstaining 5-6 days a week | 9 (40.90%) | 13 (59.09%) | 22 (22.00%) |
| Abstaining 3-4 days a week | 7 (38.88%) | 11 (61.11%) | 18 (18.00%) |
| Abstaining two or less than two days a week | 2 (6.25%) | 30 (93.43%) | 32 (32.00%) |
| Total | 42 (42.00%) | 58 (58.00%) | 100 (100%) |

As shown in the Table 4.14, out of 42 (42%) healthy respondents consuming alcohol majority i.e. 24 abstained from alcohol for more than a week. For 58 (58%) unhealthy respondents taking alcohol, majority i.e. 30 consumed alcohol almost every day. Moreover, among those (28) abstaining from alcohol for more than a week, 24

(85.71%) were healthy while for those (32) consuming alcohol almost every day, 30 (93.43%) were unhealthy.

The above data show that majority (68%) of the respondents were taking alcohol up to four days in a week and it is according to permissible limit as per WHO, while there were few respondents (32%) who were taking more than four days a week.

Also, Case 001 mentioned the intake of alcohol for four days or more in a week.

The above findings revealed that unhealthy respondents were more frequent in taking alcohol that shows the harmful effect of excess use of alcohol on the health of respondents.

***Average Number of Drinks in a Day***

As stated earlier, two standard units or less that two standard units per day do not have harmful effect on the health of a person (WHO, 1999). To identify the respondents with excess drinking habit, it is imperative to discern the consumption of number of drinks in a day by the respondents.

**Table 4.15 Distribution of Healthy/Unhealthy Respondents on the Basis of**

**Average Quantity of Alcohol Intake**

| Intake Quantity of Alcohol | Health Status | | Total |
|---|---|---|---|
| | Healthy | Unhealthy | |
| 1-2 drinks | 30 (78.94%) | 8 (21.03%) | 38 (38.00%) |
| 3-4 drinks | 11 (27.50%) | 29 (72.50%) | 40 (40.00%) |
| 5 or more drinks | 1 (4.54%) | 21 (95.45%) | 22 (22.00%) |
| Total | 42 (42.00%) | 58 (58.00%) | 100 (100%) |

Table 4.15 specifies that 30 (78.94%) healthy and 8 (21.03%) unhealthy respondents took '1-2 drinks' of alcohol, 11 (27.50%) healthy and  29 (72.50%) unhealthy respondents consumed '3-4 drinks' of alcohol, and there was 1 (4.54%) healthy and 21 (95.45%) unhealthy respondents who were taking '5 or more drinks' of alcohol.

Thus, the above data show the average number of drinks per day consumed by respondents. So, 38% of respondents were not taking more than recommended quantity of alcohol whereas rest 62% were taking more than prescribed quantity of alcohol that may be harmful for health of an individual.

Further, an increase in number of unhealthy respondents in comparison to healthy ones was observed as the quantity of alcohol consumption increases. The above findings show that alcohol consumption beyond a certain limit has negative effect on the health of an individual.

Also, in Case Study 001 it was found that doctor was consuming 3-4 drinks of alcohol at one time which is not in consonance with the WHO recommendation of ideal quantity of alcohol.

### *History of Alcohol Consumption*

History of consuming alcohol tells the number of years of consuming alcohol by a person. The possibility of harmful effect of alcohol increases with the increase in number of years of alcohol consumption. Question was asked from the 100 respondents consuming alcohol about the number of years of alcohol consumption and a comparison of healthy and unhealthy respondents was done based on it.

**Table 4.16   Distribution of Healthy/Unhealthy Respondents on the Basis of**

**History of Alcohol Consumption**

| History of Alcohol Consumption | Health Status | | Total |
|---|---|---|---|
| | Healthy | Unhealthy | |
| 0-10 years | 22 (88.00%) | 3 (12.00%) | 25 (25.00%) |
| 11-20 years | 10 (38.46%) | 16 (61.53%) | 26 (26.00%) |
| 21-30 years | 8 (29.62%) | 19 (70.37%) | 27 (27.00%) |
| 31-40 years | 2 (14.28%) | 12 (85.71%) | 14 (14.00%) |
| >40 years | 0 (0.00%) | 8 (100%) | 8 (8.00%) |
| Total | 42 (42.00%) | 58 (58.00%) | 100 (100%) |

Table 4.16 shows that around 75% of the respondents were taking alcohol for more than 10 years. Also, out of those consuming for 0-10 years, 22 (88%) were healthy and 3 (12%) were unhealthy. Those with 11-20 years of consuming alcohol, 10 (38.46%) were healthy and 16 (61.53%) were unhealthy. Those consuming alcohol

for 21-30 years, 8 (29.62%) were healthy and 19 (70.37%) were unhealthy respondents. There were 2 (14.28%) healthy and 12 (85.71%) unhealthy respondents who were drinking for 31-40 years and for those who were consuming alcohol for more than 40 years, there were no (0%) healthy and 8 (100%) unhealthy respondents i.e. all the respondents consuming alcohol for more than 40 years were unhealthy.

The above results explain that as the duration of intake of alcohol increases, the number of unhealthy respondent increases as compared to healthy respondents. So, alcohol despite having medicinal value in limited quantity if taken for a long period of time and in excess quantity has negative effect on the health of respondents.

*Change in Quantity of Consumption of Alcohol*

The doctors may increase or decrease the quantity of alcohol consumption and this may have different impact on the presence of lifestyle diseases amongst them.

**Table 4.17 Distribution of Healthy/Unhealthy Respondents on the Basis of Perception of Change in Quantity of Alcohol Consumption**

| Consumption of Alcohol | Health Status | | Total |
|---|---|---|---|
| | **Healthy** | **Unhealthy** | |
| Increased | 8 (72.72%) | 3 (27.27%) | 11 (11.00%) |
| Decreased | 3 (9.09%) | 30 (90.90%) | 33 (33.00%) |
| Remained unchanged | 31 (55.35%) | 25 (44.64%) | 56 (56.00%) |
| Total | 42 (42.00%) | 58 (58.00%) | 100 (100%) |

Table 4.17 indicates that there were 56 (56%) respondents for whom quantity of alcohol remain unchanged over the period of time. Among these 56 respondents, 31 (55.35%) were healthy and 25 (44.64%) were unhealthy, for 8 (72.72%) healthy and 3 (27.27%) unhealthy respondents, quantity had increased and for 3 (9.09%) healthy and 30 (90.90%) unhealthy respondents, quantity of alcohol had decreased.

The data show that the intake of alcohol in majority (56%) of respondents has remained the same. For those, whose intake of alcohol has increased, most of them i.e. 72.72% were healthy respondents. Also, the interesting finding is that those who had decreased their alcohol intake were mostly unhealthy i.e. around 90.90 %. This confirms that unhealthy respondents tend to reduce their alcohol intake in wake of their diseased condition.

During Focused Group Discussion, many participants remarked that if alcohol is consumed in controlled way then it has the medicinal value.

## OTHER LIFESTYLE RELATED FACTORS

Other factors related to lifestyle like sleeping habit of a person, stress in job, perception about sociality,  kind of leisure activities a person is enjoying etc. reveal a lot about the lifestyle of people and hence, possibility of falling sick. Researcher was interested to recognize all the other factors in addition to risk factors affecting the day to day life of the respondents and thus, their effect on the health of respondents.

### Sleeping Habit

According to National Heart, Lung and Blood Institute (2011), an adult's daily requirement of sleep is 7-8 hours. The lack of sleep may affect the health of an individual. Studies have found an association between lack of sleep (less than required quantity) and increase in body weight (Kohatsu et al., 2006), diabetes (Gottlieb et al., 2005), cardiovascular diseases and hypertension (Kasasbeh, Chi & Krishnaswamy, 2006).

In addition, a U-shaped relationship was established between sleep duration (both short and long) and diabetes & coronary diseases (Ayas et al., 2003) and hypertension (Gottlieb et al., 2006). Ayas et al. (2003) further added that risk for diabetes increases 1.5 times among people having short and long duration of sleep in comparison to those having normal sleep (7-8 hours).

Thus, sleep plays an important role for the overall health and well-being of an individual. Lifestyle may affect the quantity and quality of one's sleep.  Working schedule and stress may be the determining lifestyle factors affecting the sleeping habit.

So in our research, we tried to reveal this aspect of respondent's life in order to find out the number of healthy and unhealthy respondents based on their duration of sleep.

**Table 4.18 Distribution of Healthy/Unhealthy Respondents on the Basis of**

**Duration of Sleep**

| Duration of Sleep | Health Status | | Total |
|---|---|---|---|
| | **Healthy** | **Unhealthy** | |
| 7-8 hours | 35 (50.00%) | 35 (50.00%) | 70 (29.17%) |
| >8 hours | 5 (31.25%) | 11 (68.75%) | 16 (6.67%) |
| <7 hours | 70 (45.45%) | 84 (54.54%) | 154 (64.17%) |
| Total | 110 (45.83%) | 130 (54.17%) | 240 (100%) |

As shown in the Table 4.18, out of 154 (64.17%) respondents having less than 7 hours of sleep, 70 (45.45%) were healthy and 84 (54.54%) were unhealthy. Out of 70 (29.17%) respondents having 7-8 hours of sleep, number of healthy and unhealthy respondents was same i.e. 35 (50%), whereas those (6.67%) having more than 8 hours of sleep, 5 (31.25%) were healthy and 11 (68.75%) were unhealthy respondents.

The data show that most of the respondents (64.17%) were deprived of minimum required sleep of 7-8 hours. Also, there were more number of unhealthy respondents in comparison to healthy ones who had less than 7 and more than 8 hours of sleep. This illustrates that duration of sleep beyond or short of certain required duration may affect the health of an individual and results in higher number of respondents being in unhealthy condition.

**Stress in Job**

Cooper, Rout & Faragher (1989) stated that "Medical Profession is considered as high stress profession." The main reason for elevated stress in medical field is feeling of responsibility because lives of populace are involved in it (Caplan et al., 1975).

Further, there is significant relationship between long term stress in job and cardiovascular mortality. Approximately 35% of deaths due to cardiovascular diseases were due stress at work place (Johnson et al., 1996).

It is imperative to know about the healthy and unhealthy doctors' perception about stress so as to identify its effect on health.

**Table 4.19 Distribution of Healthy/Unhealthy Respondents on the Basis of**

**Perception of Stress in the Job**

| Stress in Job | Health Status | | Total |
|---|---|---|---|
| | Healthy | Unhealthy | |
| Very stressful | 15 (41.66%) | 21 (58.33%) | 36 (15.00%) |
| Moderately stressful | 65 (43.91%) | 83 (56.08%) | 148 (61.67%) |
| Not at all stressful | 30 (53.57%) | 26 (46.42%) | 56 (23.33%) |
| Total | 110 (45.83%) | 130 (54.17%) | 240 (100%) |

Data in above Table 4.19 indicate that out of total 148 (61.67%) respondents who perceived their job as 'moderately' stressful, 65 (43.91%) were healthy and 83 (56.08%) unhealthy, while for those 56 (23.33%) who said that their job is 'not at all' stressful, 30 (53.57%) were healthy and 26 (46.42%) were unhealthy respondents. Among those 36 (15%) respondents who felt that their job was 'very stressful', 15 (41.66%) were healthy and 21 (58.33%) were unhealthy.

Table 4.19 shows that for majority of respondents i.e. 184 (76.67%) the job or work was more or less stressful whereas for 56 (23.33%) the job is 'not at all' stressful.

Thus, the number of unhealthy (104) respondents was found to be higher than healthy (80) ones among 184 (76.67%) respondents for whom the job or work was 'moderately' or 'very stressful', whereas there was not much difference in number of healthy (30) and unhealthy (26) respondents who did not take their job stressful. So, stress has negative effect on the health of individuals.

Case 003, who was unhealthy, also reported stressful working conditions whereas Case 013 did not consider the work stressful and was healthy even at the age of 65 years.

In consonance with the above findings, many studies found the feeling of stressful working conditions among doctors, for instance, studies by Menon & Munalula (2007), Wond (2008), Huggard & Dixon (2011), Govender et al. (2012), Tuthill et al. (2013).

**'Sociality'**

According to 'Collin English Dictionary' (2014) "Sociality is State or quality of being sociable or tendency to associate with others." A person may have solitary or gregarious type of personal life. In solitary personal life, a person is not having much social interaction and remains satisfied by living alone but in gregarious one, the person enjoys the company of others.

'Sociality' i.e. associating with others is beneficial for the health of individuals. A number of studies show a link between social ties and health. Low social ties both in quantity and quality had negative effect on cardiovascular, endocrine and immune systems (Everson-Rose, Susan & Lewis, 2005; Robles & Kiecolt-Glasser, 2003).

In our research, we wanted to find out the respondents' perception about their 'Sociality' and its effect on their health.

**Table 4.20 Distribution of Healthy/Unhealthy Respondents on the Basis of**

**Perception about their Sociality**

| Sociality | Health Status | | Total |
|---|---|---|---|
| | Healthy | Unhealthy | |
| Solitary | 20 (30.76%) | 45 (69.23%) | 65 (27.08%) |
| Gregarious | 85 (53.13%) | 75 (46.87%) | 160 (66.67%) |
| Can not say | 5 (33.33%) | 10 (66.67%) | 15 (6.25%) |
| Total | 110 (45.83%) | 130 (54.17%) | 240 (100%) |

The data in Table 4.20 depict that out of total 160 (66.67%) respondents living gregarious life, 85 (53.13%) were healthy and 75 (46.87%) were unhealthy and for 65 (27.08%)  respondents living solitary life, 20 (30.76%) were healthy and 45 (69.23%) were unhealthy.

Further, maximum number of respondents i.e. 160 (66.67%) said that they were living a gregarious life whereas 65 (27.08%) respondents told that their life is solitary in nature.

Data show that most (69.23%) of respondents living solitary life were unhealthy whereas the number of healthy respondents (53.13%) was more in comparison to unhealthy ones (46.87%) who were living gregarious life.

In Cases 003 and 005, low social interaction was found and doctors in these case studies were suffering from hypertension and diabetes respectively. Whereas, in Case 012 doctor was very social and leading a healthy life even at the age of 62 years. This shows that low social interaction may have some negative effect on the health of a person.

Thus, gregarious type of living seems to have good effect on the health of respondents.

**Choice of Leisure Activity**

Kleiber & Nimrod (2009) defined leisure activities as "Preferred and enjoyable activities participated in during one's free time." Choice of leisure time activities is good indicator of lifestyle of the people. Some leisure activities like playing games, interacting with people, and dancing etc. indicate some extent of physical activity but activities like reading books, watching television and listening to music during leisure time point towards the sedentary lifestyle. Researcher was interested in knowing about the leisure activities among healthy and unhealthy respondents to have an insight into lifestyle of respondents.

**Table 4.21 Distribution of Healthy/Unhealthy Respondents on the Basis of Choice of Leisure activity**

| Choice of Leisure activity | Health Status | | Total* |
|---|---|---|---|
| | **Healthy** | **Unhealthy** | |
| Spending time with family | 16 (51.61%) | 15 (48.38%) | 31 (12.91%) |
| Spending time with friends and relatives | 16 (44.44%) | 20 (55.56%) | 36 (15.00%) |
| Watching T.V. | 43 (35.24%) | 79 (64.75%) | 122 (50.83%) |
| Reading books | 51 (48.11%) | 55 (51.88%) | 106 (44.16%) |
| Other activities (dancing, listening music, cooking etc.) | 19 (40.42%) | 28 (59.57%) | 47 (19.58%) |
| No time for leisure activities | 11 (52.38%) | 10 (47.61%) | 21 (8.75%) |

*Multiple Responses

As shown in the Table 4.21, majority of respondents highlighted activities like watching T.V. and reading books as their choice of leisure activities. 51 (48.11%) healthy and 55 (51.88%) unhealthy respondents preferred to read books as their leisure time activity, 43 (35.24%) healthy and 79 (64.75%) unhealthy respondents watched T.V. in their free time. In addition,   there were 11 (52.38%) healthy and 10 (47.61%) unhealthy respondents having no time for leisure activities. All the above activities indicate a sedentary lifestyle which may cause lifestyle related diseases

On the other hand, 19 (40.42%) healthy and 28 (59.57%) unhealthy respondents showed interest in other activities (dancing, listening music, cooking etc.), 16 (51.61%) healthy and 15  (48.38%) unhealthy respondents spent their free time by spending time with family, 16 (44.44%) healthy and 20 (55.56%) unhealthy respondents preferred to interact with the relative and friends in their leisure time.

From the above data, it is clear, most preferred leisure time activities were watching television and reading books whereas least preferred ones were spending time with family, friends and relatives. The sedentary leisure activities like watching T.V. and reading books were more visible in unhealthy respondents as compared to healthy respondents.

Sedentary lifestyle is considered as one of the risk factor that catalyzes the occurrence of lifestyle related diseases. During Focused Group Discussion, some of the participants told that they watched T.V. and read books in their free time.  Case no. 003 mentioned reading books and Case no. 015 reported reading books, watching television and listening to music as their leisure time activities which were sedentary in nature and may promote an unhealthy lifestyle.

**Routine Check-ups**

A check-up is defined as, "health care motivated by the need to assess general health and prevent future illness rather than to attend to symptoms" (Sox, 2013, p.2496). Screening or regular health checkups are essential for early detection of the diseases like cancers, diabetes, heart diseases and other chronic illnesses (Schmidt, 2016).

Regular medical check-ups are essential for timely diagnosis of a disease among individuals. These check-ups are even more important in unhealthy individuals to detect the latest condition and development of complications, if any, due to their chronic conditions. Therefore respondents were asked regarding the frequency of medical check-ups and a comparison was done on this basis among healthy and unhealthy respondents.

**Table 4.22   Distribution of Healthy/Unhealthy Respondents on the Basis of Frequency of Routine Overall Check-ups per Year**

| Routine Check-ups per Year | Health Status | | Total |
| --- | --- | --- | --- |
| | Healthy | Unhealthy | |
| Not at all/Irregular | 71 (72.45%) | 27 (27.55%) | 98 (40.83%) |
| Once | 30 (35.29%) | 55 (64.71%) | 85 (35.41%) |
| 2-3 times | 9 (20.93%) | 34 (79.07%) | 43 (17.91%) |
| >3 times | 0 (0.00%) | 14 (100%) | 14 (5.83%) |
| Total | 110 (45.83%) | 130 (54.17%) | 240 (100%) |

Data in the Table 4.22 show out of 240 respondents, 98 (40.83%) were irregular or not at all going for their routine health check-ups while 85 (35.41%) went for check-ups once a year. Other 43 (17.91%) respondents got it done 2-3 times in a year and only 14 (5.83%) respondents  went for health check-ups more than 3 times in a year.

Among those (98) who never went or were irregular in overall routine health check-ups, 71 (72.45%) were healthy and 27 (27.55%) were unhealthy. For those (85), who underwent overall routine check-ups once a year, 30 (35.29%) were healthy and 55 (64.71%) unhealthy respondents. For those (43), who got their routine health check-ups done 2-3 times in a year, 9 (20.93%) were healthy and 34 (79.07%) were unhealthy. Finally, among those (14) who were having regular overall routine check-ups > 3 times per year, there was no (0%) healthy and 14 (100%) unhealthy respondents.

This data show that higher number (71) of healthy respondents did not go for medical check-ups regularly and there was small number (57) among both healthy and unhealthy respondents who got their check-ups done multiple times. While among unhealthy respondents, most (64.71%) of the respondents got their medical check-up done at least once a year. Still around 27.55 % unhealthy respondents did not care to get medical checkups done even once a year, that shows the negligence on their part as 'doctor-patients'. Overall regular health check-ups were more common among the unhealthy respondents due to development of disease as compared to healthy respondents.

Absence of habit of regular check-ups was observed in case studies too. In Case Studies 001 and 003, it was observed that doctors were not regular in their health check-ups even after the development of a chronic illness, whereas in Case Studies 006 and 008, medical check-ups were done only when the symptoms of the disease appeared.

## SUMMARY

This chapter is an attempt to compare the lifestyle and risk factors among healthy and unhealthy respondents. Along with the four main risk factors like unhealthy diet, physical inactivity, consumption of tobacco and excessive use of alcohol, other lifestyle related factors have also been explored. The other lifestyle factors like sleeping habit, stress in job, regular health check-ups, perception about sociality, leisure activities etc. tell a lot about the lifestyle of respondents and consequently effect of these factors on their health.

Higher number of unhealthy respondents was living sedentary (62.26%) and moderately active life (60%) as compared to healthy respondents. However, the number of healthy respondents (81.08%) living a very active life was higher in number as compared to that of (18.92%) of unhealthy respondents living the same. This illustrates the importance of physical activity in keeping oneself healthy.

As far as the risk factors were concerned, both healthy and unhealthy respondents were evenly involved in unhealthy dietary intake. Majority of respondents (75.83%) were regular in their meal schedule and most (52.19%) of them were healthy. Among those who were taking irregular (24.16%), meal schedule, majority (74.13%) were found to be unhealthy. Busy schedule (79.31%) was the most common reason given for irregularity in meal schedule.

The findings show that both healthy and unhealthy respondents were more or less in the habit of dining outside. But frequent intake of junk food is more common among unhealthy respondents. Unhealthy respondents were taking required amount of healthy diet in the form of consumption of fruits and vegetables or legumes. It appears that unhealthy respondents began to follow a healthy lifestyle after the development of disease. Findings also revealed the trend of taking less than required quantity of milk and milk products amongst unhealthy respondents. However, healthy respondents showed less inclination towards healthy diet pattern.

Different range of unhealthy BMI, for instance, overweight, obese and severely obese was witnessed more among unhealthy respondents as compared to healthy respondents. Number of healthy respondents (52.94%) doing regular exercise were observed to be more in number as compared to unhealthy respondents (47.06%). This reflects the good effect of physical work out on the health of respondents. Busy schedule (65.38%) is assigned as the most common reason against physical activity. Most commonly performed physical activity was walking (85) and least commonly performed was swimming (7).

As far as the habit of tobacco consumption was concerned, the respondents taking tobacco products were mostly unhealthy (62.07%). This shows that consumption of tobacco products is one of the risk factors for the development of disease.

Further, number of unhealthy respondents (58%) taking alcohol was more than the healthy respondents (42%) taking alcohol. Thus alcohol consumption may be one of the factors for the causation of disease. More frequent intake of alcohol was seen more among unhealthy respondents as compared to healthy respondents. Moreover, long duration of alcohol consumption was seen to have an adverse effect on the health of individual even if consumed within limit.

As we examined the other lifestyle related factors, it was found that in case of both long (>8 hours) and short hours (<7 hours) of sleep, the number of unhealthy respondents was higher (68.75% and 54.54% respectively) in contrast to healthy ones (31.25% and 45.45% respectively). This shows that duration of sleep beyond or short of certain required duration i.e. 7-8 hours/ night results in more respondents in unhealthy condition.

Percentage of unhealthy respondents (58.33%) with perception of high stress in job was more as compared to healthy respondents (41.66%). This indicates that stress beyond a certain level has harmful effect on the health of individuals.

Effect of sociality on the health of the respondents had also been observed in the study. Solitary living was more common among unhealthy respondents (69.23%) as compared to healthy ones (30.76%) whereas respondents having a gregarious life were found to be healthy (53.13%) in comparison to unhealthy ones (46.87%). Further, the sedentary leisure activities like watching T.V. and reading books were more frequent among unhealthy respondents as compared to healthy respondents. Sedentary lifestyle is considered as one of the risk factor that catalyzes the occurrence of lifestyle related diseases.

Overall regular health check-ups were more common among the unhealthy respondents than in healthy respondents. This was perhaps due to the development of health related issues that compelled unhealthy respondents to get their routine check-ups done on regular basis. However, an overall attitude of carelessness had been witnessed in case of healthy respondents (72.45%) who didn't go for regular health check-ups.

Therefore, in the present chapter, comparison of risk factors and lifestyle among healthy and unhealthy respondents was done in order to identify the reasons for the occurrence of lifestyle related diseases. This chapter also highlighted the tendency of unhealthy respondents to follow a healthy lifestyle. Moreover, presence of risk factors among healthy respondents suggested the possibility for occurrence of these diseases amongst them.

# CHAPTER V

# IMPACT OF LIFESTYLE RELATED DISEASES ON DOCTORS

As discussed in the previous chapters, the incidence of lifestyle related diseases is quite high these days. This is happening primarily due to changed lifestyle. The risk factors like high job stress, inadequate exercise schedule, inappropriate eating habits etc. are present among doctors and result in to onset of lifestyle related diseases.

Lifestyle related diseases has long term effects on the lives of people due to their chronic nature. Livneh and Antonak (2005) established that chronic illnesses have major impact on physical, psychological and social aspects of a person's life. According to McBride (1993) and Lubkin (2005), "chronic illnesses may contribute to impaired physical functioning, limitations in activities of daily living, loss of independence, pain, emotional distress and changes in self-identity" (as cited in Whittemore & Dixon, 2008).

Hence, at physical level these diseases interrupt the day to day life of an individual by affecting a person physically through causing pain, discomfort or fatigue in the body. At social level it affects the social ties with family and friends, at the psychological level it disturbs an individual emotionally and mentally while at economic level the financial burden on the individual is increased.

Since lifestyle related diseases affect the every domain of human life, accordingly these diseases shape the lifestyle choices like diet, extent of physical activity and living environment of patient and thus, quality of life of the patient gets affected (Newman, Steed & Mulligan, 2004). Lifestyle related diseases due to their chronic condition, therefore, affect quality of life of an individual.

A person suffering from chronic illness has to maintain a balance between expectations of personal life and ailing condition. The patients may have to take regular medicines and sometimes adjust with disability due to disease for the rest of his life. So personal, social, economic and psychological cost of lifestyle related diseases is very high.

It is important to identify the impact of lifestyle diseases among doctors. So, the researcher tried to know about the perception of the doctors regarding the impact of lifestyle related diseases. There were 130 unhealthy respondents out of total sample of 240 respondents. These respondents were asked questions related to their perception about personal, social, economic and psychological impact of the lifestyle related diseases.

**IMPACT OF LIFESTYLE RELATED DISEASES ON PERSONAL LIFE**

Pesonal life of an individual includes activities related to household and outdoor tasks or responsibilities as well as eating behaviour. When a person suffers from lifestyle related diseases then his or her personal life gets affected. In this section, impact of lifestyle related diseases on the daily routine, outdoor activities and eating habits have been discussed.

**Impact on Daily/ Routine Activities**

Daily/routine activities involve a number of activities which are associated with selfcare and the care of the family. These activities are differentiated on the basis of gender and age. Long term health issues may always interfere with the daily/routine activities. For instance, Volpato et al. (2002) discussed the impact of diabetes on mobility among women and observed that there is higher incidence of mobility disability that results in to walking limitation among women with diabetes.  This limited ability inturn may affect the day to day routine activities.

To know about the effect of lifestyle related diseases on the respondents' routine activities, question was asked about the respondents' perception of impact on daily or routine activities due to these diseases.

**Table 5.1  Distribution of Respondents' Perception of Impact on Daily/Routine Activities**

| City | Impact  on Daily/Routine Activities | | | Total |
|---|---|---|---|---|
| | **Never** | **Sometimes or Moderate** | **Mostly** | |
| Patiala | 34 (61.81%) | 18 (32.72%) | 3 (5.45%) | 55 (42.30%) |
| Amritsar | 29 (38.67%) | 41 (54.66%) | 5 (6.67%) | 75 (57.69%) |
| Total | 63 (48.46%) | 59 (45.38%) | 8 (6.15%) | 130 (100%) |

Table 5.1 shows that out of 130 unhealthy respondents, 63 (48.46%) respondents said that they 'never' felt any impact on their daily/routine activities. Moreover, 59 (45.38%) felt the impact 'sometimes' and there were 8 (6.15%) respondents who reported effect of lifestyle diseases on their daily/routine activities 'mostly'.

Data depict that though 63 (48.46%) respondents felt no interference with their daily/routine activities but 67 out of 130 i.e. 51.53% respondents said that they had felt the impact of lifestyle related diseases on their daily/routine activities and this impact varied from 'sometimes' to 'mostly'.

In the Case Study 010, it was found that the disease affected the daily life of the female doctor suffering from rheumatoid arthritis. She had the feeling of stiffness and pain in her joints that interfered with her routine and household work.

During Focused Group Discussion, Dr. J suffering from arthritis said that when the physical pain due to arthritis in the body is very severe, it restricts the mobility and result in interference in her routine activities.

**Impact on Outdoor Activities**

The outdoor activities in the form of physical workout i.e. running, walking, jogging, cycling and recreational activities like going to cinema, party or shopping help in socializing with the new people and new social environment. To know about the impact of lifestyle related diseases on the outdoor activities, question was asked about the respondents' perception of the impact of disease on their outdoor activities.

Table 5.2  Distribution of Respondents' Perception of<br>Impact on Outdoor Activities

| City | Impact on Outdoor Activities | | | Total |
|------|------|------|------|------|
| | **Never** | **Sometimes or Moderate** | **Mostly** | |
| Patiala | 33 (60.00%) | 18 (32.72%) | 4 (7.27%) | 55 (42.30%) |
| Amritsar | 30 (40.00%) | 40 (53.33%) | 5 (6.67%) | 75 (57.69%) |
| Total | 63 (48.47%) | 58 (44.61%) | 9 (6.92%) | 130 (100%) |

As shown in the Table 5.2, out of total 130 unhealthy respondents, 63 (48.47%) respondents did not feel any impact on their outdoor activities like physical workout or recreational activities etc. Further, 58 (44.61%) respondents perceived 'moderate or sometimes' impact of the disease on their outdoor activities. However, 9 (6.92%) respondents felt the impact on their outdoor activities 'mostly'.

Data depict that though i.e. 63 (48.47%) respondents felt no impact of disease on their outdoor activities but a large number i.e. 67 (51.53%) respondents perceived 'moderate impact' to 'deep impact' on their outdoor activities.

A mixed impact of lifestyle related diseases on outdoor activities had also been observed in case studies. In Case Study 004, the doctor explained that there was a moderate impact on his outdoor activities after the detection of the disease. Whereas in Case Study 005, the doctor increased his recreational activities so as to deal with his problem of depression due to lifestyle related disease.

In Focused Group Discussion, Doctors mentioned that their outdoor activities got affected due to the diseases. For instance, Dr. I said that he had less inclination for going outside when sugar level is high. Further, Dr. E sometimes has to stay indoor because of pollution and dust outside to avoid the further aggravation of his asthmatic condition. Similarly, outdoor activities of Dr. J are restricted due to arthritis.

**Impact on Eating Habits**

As discussed earlier, there seems to be a clear relationship between the diet and development of lifestyle related diseases. Diet is one of modifiable behavior risk factors which can lead to causation of diseases, so in order to manage the lifestyle related diseases, one has to make changes in day to day eating habits. For example, if a patient is suffering from diabetes, he has to cut sugar intake and patient of hypertension has to eat food with less salt and oil.

Researcher was interested in knowing about the respondents' perception about impact of lifestyle related diseases on their eating habits. This can tell us about the possible change or alteration in eating habits because of onset of the lifestyle related diseases.

Table 5.3 Distribution of Respondents' Perception of Impact on<br>Routine Eating Habits

| City | Impact on Routine Eating Habits | | | Total |
|---|---|---|---|---|
| | **Never** | **Sometimes or Moderate** | **Mostly** | |
| Patiala | 7 (12.72%) | 18 (32.72%) | 30 (54.54%) | 55 (42.30%) |
| Amritsar | 8 (10.67%) | 24 (32.00%) | 43 (57.33%) | 75 (57.69%) |
| Total | 15 (11.54%) | 42 (32.31%) | 73 (56.15%) | 130 (100%) |

The Table 5.3 indicates that out of 130 unhealthy respondents, 73 (56.15%) respondents felt that lifestyle related diseases had affected their normal eating habits 'mostly', Further, 42 (32.31%) respondents remarked 'sometimes or moderate' interference, and 15 (11.54%) respondents said lifestyle related diseases 'never' had an effect on their diet and eating habits.

Thus, most of respondents i.e. (56.15%) were feeling that their eating habits had been affected to a great extent. This may be probably due to the awareness of most of the respondents that their diet should fit with their physical condition. Moreover, they also know the role of healthy eating in management of lifestyle related diseases. Therefore, the disease had impacted their eating habits and they had modified their dietary habit to reduce the impact of the disease.

Some of the Case Studies also explained how the respondents were forced to make modification in the eating habits after development of disease. In Case 006, the doctor started eating healthy home cooked food with low sodium and low fat contents after he was detected with cardiac problem. In Case Study 009, the doctor had reduced consuming junk food but not stopped to take it completely whereas in Case 001 the doctor made few changes in his eating habits.

During Focused Group Discussion, Dr. L explained how his eating habits were also very much affected due to heart problem and he was avoiding the high fat and high sodium diet. Eating habits of Dr. I, a diabetic patient, also suffered a lot. He was very fond of sweets and chocolates but now he has to stop eating these things. Also, Dr. E suffering from asthma felt that his asthmatic condition affected his eating habits.

**IMPACT OF LIFESTYLE RELATED DISEASES ON SOCIAL LIFE**

Personal life of an individual can not be isolated from his social life. If a disease affects the personal life of an individual, it may also equally affect the social life.

As we know that social life is mainly concerned with social ties with family, friends or neighbors. To know about the impact of lifestyle related diseases on social life, question was asked from respondents about their perception of impact on normal social activities with family, friends and neighbors.

Also, a feeling of 'stigma' due to lifestyle related diseases may arise in the social setup when an unhealthy person interacts with other persons in the society. In case of doctors as well the presence of feeling of any kind of stigma and their perception about the feeling of 'stigma' has been discussed in this section.

**Social Activities with Family, Friends and Neighbors**

Lifestyle related diseases once occurred, they cannot be cured completely. These diseases can interfere with normal social activities of the patients with their family, friends, or neighbors. Royer (1998) explored the impact of chronic disease on the social interaction and found that due to chronic illness social interactions become lessened and impaired and that result in to social isolation.

Question was asked from 130 unhealthy respondents about their perception of interference with their social activities in order to identify the impact of disease on social life.

**Table 5.4 Distribution of Respondents' Perception of Impact on**

**Normal Social Activities with Family, Friends or Neighbors**

| City | Impact on Normal Social Activities | | | Total |
|------|------|------|------|------|
| | **Never** | **Sometimes** | **Mostly** | |
| Patiala | 30 (54.54%) | 23 (41.81%) | 2 (3.63%) | 55 (42.30%) |
| Amritsar | 32 (42.67%) | 38 (50.66%) | 5 (6.67%) | 75 (57.69%) |
| Total | 62 (47.69%) | 61 (46.92%) | 7 (5.38%) | 130 (100%) |

Data shown in Table 5.4 highlight the respondents' perception of impact caused by lifestyle related diseases on normal social activities. Out of total 130 unhealthy respondents suffering from lifestyle related diseases, 62 (47.69%) respondents felt that their normal social activities were 'never' affected by their health condition whereas 61 (46.92%) respondents said that their social activities were affected 'sometimes' and  7 (5.38%) respondents told that their normal social activities were affected 'mostly' due to their diseased condition.

Data depict that though 62 (47.69%) respondents perceived no interference of disease with their normal social activities, but 68 (52.30%) respondents out of 130 respondents felt an impact on their social activities from 'sometimes' to 'mostly'.

From the data, it appears that more than half of the respondents (68) because of their ill health felt the disturbance in social life.  But there were large numbers of respondents (62) who did not feel any impact on their social life. This may be due to their better management of lifestyle related diseases as compared to others who felt interference.

In case studies, some doctors said that their social activities had been affected a lot e.g. doctors in Case Studies 001,009, 010, 016 whereas some others in Case Studies 003, 004, 008, 017 reported that they had negligible or moderate effect on their social activities.  Importantly, in Case Study 005 the doctor said that he increased his social activities to cope up with the anxiety caused after the detection of diabetes.

In Focused Group Discussion, Dr. H, a survivor of cervical cancer, explained how her social activities were restricted initially during the course of treatment but afterwards she was having the normal social activities.

**'Stigma' due to  lifestyle related diseases.**

Concept of 'Stigma' is becoming a focus of attention among the health professionals as well as among common people. Stigma has become an area of interest in public health because it is becoming a prominent feature of a number of chronic diseases. It has now been recoganized as an important component of social impact of disease (Weiss, Ramakrishna & Somma, 2006).

Goffman (1963) conceptualized the concept of stigma as, "the situation of the individual who is disqualified from full social acceptance." In contemporary society the persons suffering from communicable chronic diseases like AIDS, STDs, skin diseases and mental illness are sometimes not accepted as normal persons and they may feel stigmatized due to their disease.

Feeling of stigma due to chronic illness often makes a person feel hesitant about revealing any health related problem to other people. This may be because he/she considers the disease as a blot on his/her image.

Doctors are always considered as 'care givers'. It may be uncomfortable for them to be in a position of 'care taker'. So, a sense of stigma may prevail in some situations.

Researcher was thus interested in knowing whether doctors suffering from lifestyle related diseases feel a sense of stigma due to their physical illness or not.

So, question was asked about the feeling of stigma due to lifestyle related diseases.

**Table 5.5 Distribution of Respondents on the Basis of Perception of**

**Feeling of Stigma**

| City | Feeling of Stigma | | | Total |
|---|---|---|---|---|
| | **Never** | **Sometimes** | **Mostly** | |
| Patiala | 52 (94.54%) | 3 (5.45%) | 0 (0.00%) | 55 (42.30%) |
| Amritsar | 68 (90.67%) | 7 (9.33%) | 0 (0.00%) | 75 (57.69%) |
| Total | 120 (92.30%) | 10 (7.69%) | 0 (0.00%) | 130 (100%) |

Table 5.5 shows that majority of respondents i.e. 120 (92.30%) out of total 130 unhealthy respondents, had never felt any stigma due to lifestyle related disease. Out of these 120 respondents who had no feeling of stigma, 52 (94.54%) respondents belonged to Patiala and 68 (90.67%) were from Amritsar. Out of 10 (7.69%) respondents feeling the stigma 'sometimes', 3 (5.45%) were from Patiala and 7 (9.33%) were from Amritsar. There were no respondent who had feeling of stigma 'mostly' or frequently.

The above given information shows majority (92.30%) of respondents did not consider chronic illness or disease as stigma. The reason may be that in contemporary times, the lifestyle related diseases are the most common type of diseases among people. So, onset of such diseases is no more a stigma nowadays as compared to mental illness and other communicable diseases. Communicable diseases such as AIDS, skin diseases etc., however, result in stigma.

In most of the Case Studies and Focused Group Discussion, no respondent explicitly reported the feeling of stigma due to the diseased condition.   However, in the Case 001, doctor felt that social interaction has reduced a lot as people avoid him because they don't like to  interact with an unhealthy person.

## ECONOMIC IMPACT OF LIFESTYLE RELATED DISEASES

Along with the impact of lifestyle related diseases on personal and social lives, the researcher was also interested in knowing about economic aspects and impact of lifestyle related diseases on the unhealthy respondents. Economic impact tells whether the person has any increased economic burden due to his or her disease.   In general, the treatment for lifestyle related diseases extends for a long period of time and in modern days health care is very expensive. A lot of money has to spend on the treatment of these diseases. The treatment involves intake of medicine, periodic medical tests or examinations and routine visits to doctors. This leads to increase in economic burden on the individual suffering from lifestyle related diseases.

Researcher was particularly interested in knowing about the economic impact of lifestyle related diseases on doctors.  The doctors are considered to be the quite well off section of the society economically. So, it was considered important to know the perception of the doctors towards the direct or indirect cost of lifestyle related Diseases.

Here, economic aspects and impact of  of lifestyle related diseases on the respondents has been noticed in two ways:

a) Direct cost of lifestyle related diseases

b) Indirect cost of lifestyle related diseases

### a)    Direct Cost of Lifestyle related Diseases

Direct cost is concerned with the direct expenditure on the disease in terms of expenditure on medicines, medical tests, hospitalization of patient etc. Researcher was interested in knowing the perception of respondents about the economic effect of lifestyle related diseases. So, question was asked from 130 unhealthy respondents related to this subject.

**Table 5.6 Distribution of Respondents on the Basis Perception of**

**Direct Cost of Lifestyle related Diseases**

| City | Direct Cost of Lifestyle related Diseases | | | Total |
|---|---|---|---|---|
| | **Very less/Not at all** | **Moderately** | **Very much** | |
| Patiala | 44 (80.00%) | 11 (20.00%) | 0 (0.00%) | 55 (42.30%) |
| Amritsar | 64 (85.33%) | 11 (14.67%) | 0 (0.00%) | 75 (57.69%) |
| Total | 108 (83.07%) | 22 (16.92%) | 0 (0.00%) | 130 (100%) |

Table 5.6 gives the information about the direct economic cost of lifestyle related diseases. Out of total 130 unhealthy respondents suffering from lifestyle related diseases, 108 (83.07%) respondents felt no or very less economic impact while 22 (16.92%) felt 'moderate' economic impact and there was no (0%) respondent who felt that the economic impact of the disease 'very much'

The data show that majority of the respondents i.e. 108 (83.07%) felt no or very less economic effect of disease. The reason behind feeling not much economic burden of the disease may be that doctors are mostly from upper middle class families. Also, medical profession is a well-paid profession and doctors are earning a good amount of money. So, they are very much in a position to afford the expenditure on their health related problems comfortably. In some cases they get health care from the hospital where they are working in free or discounted rates.

*Managing Expenses of Disease*

Above given data revealed that doctors are not very much affected by the economic burden of the disease. However, it is imperative to know how they managed the expenses when some kind of health related problem was faced by them. Question was asked from the respondents whether they manage the expenditure by health insurance, medical reimbursement in case of government job, out of pocket expenditure or by other sources like samples, medicine on low rates etc.

**Table 5.7 Distribution of Respondents on the Basis of**

**Managing Expenses of Disease**

| City | Managing Expenses of Disease | | | | Total |
|---|---|---|---|---|---|
| | **Health Insurance** | **Reimbursement** | **Out of Pocket** | **Other Sources** | |
| Patiala | 3 (5.45%) | 3 (5.45%) | 41(74.54%) | 8(14.54%) | 55(42.30%) |
| Amritsar | 0 (0.00%) | 3 (4.00%) | 72 96.00%) | 0 (0.00%) | 75(57.69%) |
| Total | 3 (2.30%) | 6 (4.61%) | 113(86.92%) | 8 (6.15%) | 130 (100%) |

Table 5.7 depicts that majority of the doctors i.e. 113 (86.92%) met the expenses of disease on their own whereas 8 (6.15%) respondents mentioned the other sources to meet their expenses. Further, 6 (4.61%) and 3 (2.30%) respondents met their medical expenses through medical reimbursement and health insurance respectively.

Majority of the respondents i.e. 113 (86.92%) according to above given data managed their expenses from their own pocket

During Focused Group Discussion, nearly all the doctors mentioned that due to their well to do life, the economic impact is less evident than the social and personal impacts.

This shows the good economic condition of the doctors as they were able to spend money on treatment of their illness.

**b) Indirect Cost of Lifestyle related Diseases**

Indirect cost of illness is measured by loss of income due to being absent or taking break from work and effect on the efficiency of work (Koopmanschap, Burdorf & Lötters, 2013). When a person suffers from a chronic illness then there is possibility that professional life of that person may suffer.

***Break from Work***

Suffering from lifestyle related diseases sometimes make it difficult for doctors to work properly. So, doctors sometimes have to take break from work to manage their health related issues. Also, break from work brings with it a loss of income for the doctors especially for those who are in private practice. Due to this poor health condition, person may take break from professional life for some time that may result in loss of income.

### *Effect on Efficiency of Work*

Lerner et al. (2003) discussed about the probability of productivity loss at the work place due to chronic health condition. Further, Burton et al. (2004) observed that both acute and chronic health conditions are linked with the loss in productivity at work place. When a person suffers from a disease for a long duration of time then efficiency and productivity gets affected and  hence income at the work place may be impinged on. Doctors are not an exception to it.

In order to know the indirect cost of diseases, a question was asked from the unhealthy respondents to know about the effect of chronic illness on the  efficiency of work and the losses due to break in work.

**Table 5.8 Distribution of Respondents' on the Basis of Perception Regarding Indirect Cost of Lifestyle related Diseases**

| Indirect Cost | Never | Sometimes | Mostly | Total |
|---|---|---|---|---|
| Losses due to Break from Work | 47 (36.15%) | 71(54.61%) | 12(9.23%) | 130(100%) |
| Effect on the Efficiency of Work | 65 (50.00%) | 61(46.92%) | 4 (3.07%) | 130(100%) |

As shown in Table 5.8, there were 71 (54.61%) unhealthy respondents who said that they had to suffer economic losses 'sometimes' as a result of taking break due to illness, 47 (36.15%) 'never' experienced loss of income due to illness, and 12 (9.23%) respondents told that they had income loss  'mostly' during illness. The data specified that most of the unhealthy respondents i.e. 71 (54.61%)  said that they had economic losses due to break from work during illness but break from work was not too frequent. There were 36.15% respondents who did not have loss of income due to their chronic health issues.

Case Studies 006 and 016 are peculiar because Case 006 suffering from cardiac problem and Case 016 (working as gynaecologist) suffering from hypertension, mild osteoarthritis, and depression had losses due to taking break from work.

Further, it is clear from the Table 5.8 that out of total 130 unhealthy respondents, 65 (50%) respondents never felt an effect on the efficiency of work due to illness, 61 (46.92%) respondents felt its effect on the efficiency of work for 'sometimes', only 4 (3.07%)  had the feeling of effect on the efficiency of work 'mostly'. This data show that 50% of respondents felt that lifestyle related diseases affected the efficiency of work. So, it implies that chronic health issues more or less affect the efficiency of work and have a negative effect on the professional growth of the 'doctor-patient'. However, there were equal numbers of respondents who considered that lifestyle related diseases had no effect on the efficiency of their work.  In Case 004, the doctor feels that his efficiency at work has been affected due to his chronic illness.

Doctors are considered as the elite section of the society. The medical profession is considered as the rewarding profession as far as the material gain is concerned.. The data implies that doctors are least affected economically by the lifestyle related diseases as far as the direct cost of disease is concerned. This may be due to their sound financial position, their close contacts with the other medical professionals, availability of free samples of medicine and availability of medicine at much lower rates as compared to market prices etc.

But in case of indirect cost of disease, some impact of lifestyle related diseases have been observed on doctors as far as the taking break from work or effect on efficiency of work is concerned. Due to the physical and mental exertion because of their disease, they have to take break from the work and due to break they have to suffer a loss in their income.  Lifestyle related diseases due to their chronic and long term effect ultimately affect the efficiency of their work. So, it also leads to loss in income at the professional level.

**PSYCHOLOGICAL IMPACT OF LIFESTYLE RELATED DISEASES**

Lifestyle related diseases can affect the psychological well-being of the sufferer. Turner and Kelly (2000) mentioned that change in lifestyle and long term treatment due to chronic diseases leads to emotional traumas among the sufferer. Further,

Walker (2007) mentioned that onset of chronic illness causes psychological distress and unhappiness that lowers the quality of life.

Thus, lifestyle related diseases may affect the individuals psychologically by influencing the overall mental health of an individual. These diseases may disturb the thought process of the individuals. Sometimes persons suffering from diseases do not accept the ailing condition and may deny their poor health status or sometimes they do not want to reveal their true health status. Moreover, a feeling of worry, frustration, fearfulness etc. may develop among people suffering from lifestyle related diseases.

So, after discussing the impact of lifestyle related diseases on the personal, social and economic domain of an individual, the researcher was interested in knowing the psychological impact of lifestyle related diseases on unhealthy respondents. The psychological impact can be recoganized by exploring the perception of unhealthy respondents about their quality of health and feelings of distress during this period.

**Perception about Quality of their Health**

Self-perception about quality of health means the revelation of an individual about his health. It is normally expected that healthy respondents may perceive their quality of health as excellent, fair etc. whereas unhealthy respondents may have a feeling of poor or fair for their health status. So, to discern the perception about quality of health, question was asked from 130 unhealthy respondents.

**Table 5.9 Distribution of Respondents on the Basis of Perception about**

**Quality of their Health**

| Quality of Health | Number of Respondents | Percentage |
|---|---|---|
| Excellent | 35 | 26.92% |
| Fair | 32 | 24.61% |
| Poor | 63 | 48.46% |
| Total | 130 | 100% |

Table 5.9 shows that out of total 130 unhealthy respondents, 35 (26.92%) told that their health was 'excellent', and 32 (24.61%) said it to be 'fair' and 63 (48.46%) felt that their health was 'poor'.

Data indicate that most of the respondents i.e. 67 (51.53%) said that their health was 'excellent' or 'fair' whereas significant number of respondents i.e. 63 (48.46%) respondents percieved their health as poor. It appears that the unhealthy respondents stating their health status as excellent or fair, either wanted to conceal their actual health status or they are optimistic about their health despite illness.

It is relevant to mentions here the study by Gautam and MacDonald (2001) where they observed that it is hard for doctors to accept that they have some health issue.

**Distressed Feelings Percieved During Illness**

Various types of distressed feelings may come to the mind of a person after falling ill. A feeling of frustration may come to him/her sometimes, at other time he may feel discouraged and also a feeling of fearfulness or worry for the future health may come. Due to these feelings, he/she may also feel some mental fatigue. For Instance, people suffering from diabetes (Type 2) have emotional distress that involves the feelings of frustration, discouragement, depression etc. (Polonsky et al., 1995).

The researcher was interested to know that how the doctors feel when they suffer from lifestyle related diseases. The information about the psychological impact of lifestyle related diseases on the respondents was obtained by asking questions related to the respondents' perception about the presence of distressed feeling of frustration, discouragement, fearfulness, worry, mental fatigue etc. due to their long term health issues.

**Table 5.10 Distribution of Respondents on the Basis of Distressed**

**Feelings Perceived During Illness**

| Perception of Distressed Feelings | Number of Respondents | Percentage |
|---|---|---|
| Never | 44. | 33.85% |
| Sometimes | 70 | 53.85 % |
| Mostly | 16 | 12.30% |
| Total | 130 | 100% |

As shown in the Table 5.10, out of total 130 unhealthy respondents, 44 (33.85%) respondents 'never' had distressed feelings, 70 (53.85%) felt these feelings 'sometimes' and rest 16 (12.30%) said that they had feelings of distress 'mostly'. Thus, data indicate that most (66.15%) of the respondents had the distressed feelings due to the presence of illness.

Psychological impact of lifestyle related diseases has been reported in a number of case studies. In some case studies, there was a feeling of frustration or worry or some other cases experienced a feeling of fearfulness, discouragement or mental fatigue or mixture of two or more feelings.

In Case Study 001, the doctor revealed that he was very much frustrated and fearful due to heart disease whereas in Case 002 there was feeling of discouragement and fearfulness.

However, in Case 003, there was mixed feelings of fearfulness, worry, frustration, and discouragement. Initially even the doctor in Case 007 was slightly discouraged and fearful. Further, in Case Studies 008, 009, 010, 017 the psychological impact of lifestyle related diseases was observed.

In the Focused Group Discussion, Dr. H, a cancer survivor, was very much anxious, fearful and worried about her illness especially in the initial stages of development of disease. Similarly, Doctor L felt sometimes a sense of insecurity about his future. He felt anxiety, restlessness and stress frequently. Also, Dr. J suffering from arthritis felt emotionally disturbed and depressed due to her ailing condition. However, Dr. I suffering from diabetes felt not much psychological impact as he had a family history of diabetes and he very well knew that how to manage this chronic condition.

During the Focused Group discussion, there was a general consensus that doctors are well aware of the long term effect of lifestyle related diseases and side effects of continuous use of medication on the human body. Therefore, doctors become fearful and worried about their future health when they suffer from some chronic disease.

Above findings can be related to the studies by Mckevitt & Morgan (1997) and Thompson et al. (2001) where doctors felt a feeling of guilt and embarrassment due to diseases.

**SUMMARY**

Impact of lifestyle related diseases on personal and social lives as well as on psychological and economic conditions of doctors have been discussed in this chapter. Impact of lifestyle related diseases on personal life had been observed in terms of impact on daily/routine life, outdoor activities and eating habits of respondents.

The data revealed the effect of these diseases on the routine or daily life and outdoor activities had not been felt by many people (48.46% and 48.47% respectively) and rest of the respondents reported frequent or moderate interference with routine and outdoor activities. It is important to mention that the eating habits of majority of the respondents i.e. nearly 88% of respondents had been affected by these diseases 'mostly' or 'sometimes'.

Social impact includes interference with social and family ties and development of a feeling of 'stigma'. The data related to impact of lifestyle related diseases on social life revealed that more than half (52.30%) of the respondents reported interference of their health condition with their social ties with family, friends and neighbor. However, majority (92.30%) of respondents showed no feeling of stigma due to disease.

Economic impact of the lifestyle related diseases had not been seen much as far as the direct cost of the disease was concerned due to good economic condition of doctors. Only 16.92% of respondents talked about the moderate economic impact. Majority (86.92%) of the doctors paid for their medical expenses out of their pocket. In case of indirect cost of disease, an economic loss due to break from work was suffered by most (54.61%) of respondents but not too frequently while effect on the efficiency of work was felt by half number (50%) of the respondents.

Doctors mostly show an attitude of denial for their health issue. Besides, different types of distressed feelings like fearfulness, worry, discouragement, frustration and mental fatigue were reported by most (66.15%) of the respondents.

Therefore, lifestyle related diseases influenced every sphere of human life of the respondents whether personal, social, economic or psychological condition.

# CHAPTER VI

# LIFESTYLE RELATED DISEASES AMONG DOCTORS:

# EXPERIENCES AND COPING MECHANISM

As stated in the previous chapter, chronic diseases disturb the routine life as well as the social, economic and psychological wellbeing of an individual. In view of the fact that lifestyle related diseases are of long duration, slow progression and mostly incurable, so chronic conditions once developed remain as such for the rest of life. A person passes through a variety of experiences due to these diseases. Also, management of lifestyle related diseases is a multi-dimensional and difficult task and different types of coping strategies are followed by the diseased person in this situation.

Since this study is concerned with the exploration of lifestyle related diseases among doctors, the experiences may be looked in to from two perspectives i.e. from the perspective of 'doctor-patient' and from the perspective of physician of 'doctor-patient'.

In the present chapter, thus, focus is upon the experiences and coping mechanism adopted by respondents while suffering from lifestyle related disease. The chapter is divided into two parts. The first part deals with the experiences of doctor as patient and physician of 'doctor-patient'. The second part of the chapter describes the coping mechanism adopted by the 'doctor-patients' to deal with the ailing condition.

**I**

When a doctor suffers from some chronic illness, there arises a situation of role reversal. In this state, the doctor who is normally seen in the status of health care service provider becomes the consumer of the same. A situation of role ambiguity is faced by physician and 'doctor-patient' at two different levels i.e. at the level of 'doctor-patient' as well as the physician of a 'doctor-patient' (Jaye and Wilson, 2003). Experiences in two diagonally opposite statuses may totally differ from each other as both the statues have altogether different roles to perform.

**EXPERIENCES OF 'DOCTOR-PATIENTS'**

Experiences of 'doctor-patients' had been looked in to with the help of information collected about the type of feeling on detection of disease, consultation behavior, and perception about the behavior of physician during treatment, dilemmas about taking treatment etc. This information may help us to completely understand the experiences of 'doctor-patients' while passing through illness period.

**'Feeling' on the Detection of Disease**

In the study, the first inclination was to know the perception of the respondents about their feeling on the detection of their illness i.e. whether they felt normal or disturbed on the diagnosis of disease. This may help us to find out whether the patient was able to manage the ailing condition easily or not. Question was asked from 130 unhealthy respondents to know about their feeling on detection of lifestyle related disease.

**Table 6.1 Distribution Based on Respondents' Perception about Feeling on the**

**Detection of Lifestyle related Disease**

| City | Feeling on the Detection of Disease | | Total |
|------|---------|----------|-------|
| | **Normal** | **Disturbed** | |
| Patiala | 35 (63.63%) | 20 (36.36%) | 55 (42.30%) |
| Amritsar | 43 (57.33%) | 32 (42.67%) | 75 (57.69%) |
| Total | 78 (60.00%) | 52 (40.00%) | 130 (100%) |

The Table 6.1 shows that out of 130 unhealthy respondents, 78 (60%) respondents felt 'normal' whereas 52 (40%) respondents said that they got 'disturbed' when they came to know about their disease.

According to above data, most number of respondents (60%) felt 'normal' whereas a significant number of respondents (40%) got 'disturbed' when they came to know about their illness.

In Case Studies 002, 004, 006, 009, 010 it was found that 'doctor-patients' were disturbed on diagnosis of disease while the doctors in other cases took their illness normally.

In case of the 60% doctors it seems that may be due to their professional socialization to manage the stressful circumstances and their medical understanding of the disease, they took the disease 'normally'.

However, there were doctors (40%) who got disturbed when the disease was disclosed to them. It is relevant to mention here the study of Gautam and MacDonald (2001) where they found doctors always have a denial attitude in accepting the health problem. This shows that doctors are not taking health related issues normally.

***Feeling of Disturbance***

There can never be a pleasant situation for the person who is diagnosed with a chronic illness. A person experiences distressed emotions of different intensity. The 'feeling of disturbance' brings feelings may be shock (surprised and upset), apprehension (anxiety about bad outcomes)., depression (feeling of severe despondency and rejection) or The type of response may be the indicator that how 'doctor-patients' reacted to a situation related to their health. Question was asked about the type of disturbed feeling from 52 respondents who reported a feeling of disturbance on the detection of their chronic illness.

**Table 6.2   Distribution of Respondents' Perception about Type of Disturbed Feeling on Detection of Lifestyle related Disease**

| City | Type of Disturbed Feeling | | | Total |
|------|---------|--------------|-----------|-------|
|      | **Shocked** | **Apprehensive** | **Depressed** | |
| Patiala | 6 (30.00%) | 9 (45.00%) | 5 (25.00%) | 20 (38.46%) |
| Amritsar | 12 (37.50%) | 15 (46.87%) | 5 (15.62%) | 32 (61.53%) |
| Total | 18 (34.61%) | 24 (46.15%) | 10 (19.23%) | 52 (100%) |

Table 6.2 indicates that 52 respondents out of 130 unhealthy respondents had different types of disturbed feelings like shock, apprehension and depression on detection of their health related problem. Out of 52 respondents, 24 (46.15%) respondents felt apprehensive towards their future health, 18 (34.61%) respondents felt shocked and

10 (19.23%) respondents had the feeling of depression when they were diagnosed with some kind of lifestyle related disease.

Thus, it is important to note that out of a total 130 unhealthy respondents, 52 of the respondents expressed shock, apprehension and depression on knowing about the health problem.  In Case Studies 002 and 010, the 'doctor-patients' were shocked on detection of their chronic conditions (hypertension and rheumatoid arthritis respectively) at a very young age. Further, in Case Study 006, the 'doctor-patient' found it very hard to digest the reality of his chronic disease and had mixed feelings of shock, disbelief, depression.

Also, in Case Study 009,  the doctor was taken aback when he was detected with heart disease as he had no family history of cardiac problem and in Case Study 004, the 'doctor-patient'  was very depressed on detection of a chronic health problem.

In Focused Group discussion, some of the doctors like Dr. H, Dr. L and Dr. J told that they were emotionally disturbed on detection of their disease whereas Dr. I took his chronic disease of diabetes normally.

Above findings can be corroborated with the study by Mckevitt & Morgan (1997) that reported a feeling of guilt and embarrassment both in case of acute and chronic physical illness among physicians.

**Consultation Behavior of 'Doctor-Patient'**

When a person suffers from any health related problem, he/she is expected to seek advice of a specialist for the treatment of disease.  Since the doctors have knowledge about the diseases and their treatment, they may have the tendency to self medicate themselves. Therefore, in the study, the researcher was interested in knowing the consultation behavior of 'doctor-patient'.

Consultation behavior in this study includes the information about whether 'doctor-patients' consulted a specialist for the treatment of their disease or self-medicated themselves.  It was also asked whether the consulted specialist was familiar or unfamiliar to the 'doctor-patient'  and if familiar, the type of relationship they shared between them.  The data may tell that whether the 'doctor-patient' was comfortable in discussing the health related problem and taking treatment from familiar specialist or not.

*Consulted Physician/Self Medicated*

As doctors have knowledge about the medicines available for diseases, sometimes they prefer to take medicine on their own instead of consulting some specialist. The question was asked   from unhealthy respondents to identify the habit of consulting some physician or self-medication.

**Table 6.3 Distribution of Respondents on the Basis of Consultation of Treatment**

| City | Consultation of Treatment | | Total |
| --- | --- | --- | --- |
| | **Consulted Physician** | **Self-medicated** | |
| Patiala | 43 (78.18%) | 12 (21.81%) | 55 (42.30%) |
| Amritsar | 53 (70.67%) | 22 (29.33%) | 75 (57.69%) |
| Total | 96 (73.84%) | 34 (26.15%) | 130 (100%) |

As shown in the Table 6.3, there were 96 (73.84%) unhealthy respondents who consulted some physician for the treatment of their illness and 34 (26.15%) respondents practiced self-medication.  Out of total 96 respondents who consulted some specialist, 53 (70.67%) were from Amritsar and 43 (78.18%) were from Patiala. Among those who self-medicated, 22 (29.33%) respondents were from Amritsar and 12 (21.81%) respondents were from Patiala.

It is evident from the above data that majority (73.84%) of the unhealthy respondents consulted some physician rather than treating their illness on their own.

In Case Study 006, the doctor went to see a specialist when he experienced chest pain whereas in Case Study 014, the doctor self medicated himself when he was having problem of blurred vision and redness in his eyes.

In Focused Group Discussion also the doctors pointed out that it is always better to consult a specialist as only a specialist can differentiate between a minor health related issue and emergency situation. Dr. L, Dr. J and Dr. K said that they preferred to visit a doctor to address their health related issues but Dr. I self medicated when he was diagnosed with diabetes.

Findings of some studies are not in consonance with the findings of present research, for instance, findings by Laskari et al. (2010) on the young Greek doctors, Montgomery et al. (2011) in physicians and medical students and Schulz et al. (2016) pointed towards the high rates of self-treatment among doctors.

### *Familiarity with the Consultant*

Generally, a patient consults practitioner or physician when he or she needs medical advice or care. The selection of physician may be explicit as well as implicit. In explicit choice of physician, there is an open and wider option where the patient may consult a physician according to his or her convenience. But in implicit choice, the patient seeks advice from the same physician or depends very much on the recommendations of family and friends without thinking about some another option for taking treatment and thus has limited choice (Harris, 2003).

The doctors as patients may choose the physicians for treatment on the basis of their familiarity to them. As already said that most of the unhealthy respondents (96) preferred to go to some specialist rather than opting for self-medication, so it was desired to know consultation behavior of 'doctor-patient' regarding familiarity with the physician.

**Table 6.4 Distribution of Respondents on the Basis of Preference for Familiar/ Unfamiliar Physician for Treatment**

| City | Preference for Physician | | Total |
|------|--------|----------|-------|
|      | **Familiar** | **Unfamiliar** |       |
| Patiala | 29 (67.44%) | 14 (32.55%) | 43 (44.79%) |
| Amritsar | 17(32.07%) | 36 (67.92%) | 53 (55.20%) |
| Total | 46 (47.91%) | 50 (52.08%) | 96 (100%) |

Table 6.4 specifies that out of 96 unhealthy respondents, who consulted some specialist for their treatment, 50 (52.08%) respondents preferred unfamiliar specialist and 46 (47.91%) respondents' preference was for familiar specialist.

Thus this data revealed that more numbers of respondents i.e. 50 (52.08%) were preferring an unfamiliar professional in discussing their health related issue and taking treatment rather than a familiar professional.

In Focused Group Discussion, most of the doctors preferred to consult their familiar doctor as it could save their time whereas Dr. L and Dr. F were of the views that doctor-patient relationship should not bother about familiarity but consult the professional.

### *Type of Familiarity with the Physician*

Our next interest was to know the type of familiarity a respondent shares with the consultant. Question was asked to know that for whom the respondents had preference i.e. friend, colleague or relative for taking treatment.

**Table 6.5 Distribution of Respondents on the Basis of Type of**

**Familiarity with the Physician**

| City | Type of Familiarity with the Physician | | | Total |
| --- | --- | --- | --- | --- |
| | Friend | Colleague | Relative | |
| Patiala | 8 (27.58%) | 20 (68.96%) | 1 (3.44%) | 29 (63.04%) |
| Amritsar | 7 (41.17%) | 8 (47.05%) | 2 (11.76%) | 17 (36.95%) |
| Total | 15 (32.60%) | 28 (60.86%) | 3 (6.52%) | 46 (100%) |

Table 6.5 specifies that out of 46 unhealthy respondents who consulted some familiar specialist for their treatment, 28 (60.86%) respondents consulted their colleagues, 15 (32.60%) respondents preferred treatment from a friend and 3 (6.52%) respondents consulted relative in medical profession for the diagnosis and treatment of their illness.

Data show that colleagues were most preferred (60.86%) and relatives were least preferred (6.52%) while consulting the specialist. The reason for the same may be that respondents wanted to maintain confidentiality of their health issue from close relations like friends and relatives.

**Perception about the Behavior of 'Physician' During Treatment**

The behavior of 'physician' plays an important role during the treatment of a 'doctor-patient'. Good behavior of physician gives satisfaction to the patient and helps in faster recovery from disease. Perception about behavior of 'Physician' during treatment can be measured by making out that whether the 'doctor-patient' is satisfied with the treatment or not.

*Satisfaction with the Behavior of Physician*

Shabbir, Malik & Malik (2016) and Asif et al. (2019) specified that quality of healthcare services and patient satisfaction is closely related. Therefore, quality in health care is measured by the patient's satisfaction with treatment. Enhanced patient satisfaction, in turn, related to the improved levels of observing the treatment schedule and suggested prevention as well as better clinical outcomes (Price et al., 2014). So, the question was asked whether the respondents were satisfied or not with the treatment by physicians. This may help in assessing not only the quality of health care services but also give insight in to the alignment with the treatment process and thus, possibility of quick recovery.

**Table 6.6 Distribution of Respondents on the Basis of Perception about**

**Satisfaction with Behavior of Physician**

| City | Behavior of Physician | | Total |
|------|--------------|----------------|-------|
| | **Satisfactory** | **Unsatisfactory** | |
| Patiala | 36 (83.72%) | 7 (16.27%) | 43 (44.79%) |
| Amritsar | 44 (83.01%) | 9 (16.98%) | 53 (55.20%) |
| Total | 80 (83.33%) | 16 (16.67%) | 96 (100%) |

The data in Table 6.6 show that out of total 96 unhealthy respondents who had consulted some specialist, 80 (83.33%) respondents perceived the physician's behavior as satisfactory whereas 16 (16.67%) respondents found physician's behavior unsatisfactory during treatment.

In Patiala, 36 (83.72%) respondents were satisfied and 7 (16.27%) were dissatisfied whereas in Amritsar 44 (83.01%) respondents were satisfied and 9 (16.98%) were dissatisfied. Data show that the majority of respondents i.e. 80 (83.33%) were satisfied with the behavior of doctors treating them.

The studies by Wong and Lee (2006) and Mahato and Suman (2013) highlighted the importance of satisfaction in doctor-patient relationship for the favorable results in recovery from disease during treatment.

*Reasons for Satisfaction*

Further, the respondents (80) were asked about the reasons for their satisfaction with the behavior of the physician. They were asked to reveal the most important reason for their satisfaction.

**Table 6.7 Distribution of Respondents on the Basis of Reasons for**

**Satisfaction with Treatment by the Physician**

| Most Important Reason Cited for Satisfaction | Number of respondents | Percentage |
|---|---|---|
| Priority in appointment | 15 | 18.75% |
| Free of cost treatment | 10 | 12.50% |
| Problem was taken seriously in first visit | 22 | 27.50% |
| Complete health examination was done | 15 | 18.75% |
| Comfortable in disclosing the health related problem | 18 | 22.50% |
| Total | 80 | 100% |

The data in Table 6.7 indicate that out of total 80 unhealthy respondents who were asked to tell about the most important reason for their satisfaction with the behaviour of the physician, 22 (27.50%) respondents stated that their health related problem was taken seriously in first visit. Other 18 (22.50%) respondents revealed that they were comfortable in disclosing their illness. Moreover, 15 (18.75%) respondents answered that their complete health examination was done, other 15 (18.75%) respondents cited priority in appointment as the most important reason for their satisfaction. Finally, 10 (12.50%) respondents assigned free of cost treatment by physician as the most important reason for their satisfaction.

Thus the most common reason (27.50%) for satisfaction with the behavior of the physicians was that their ailing condition was dealt with priority and seriousness. This may be due to the fact that the doctors give priority to their colleagues in terms of appointment. As colleagues and co-workers from same profession, their problem was taken seriously and they were comfortable in disclosing and discussing their health related issues with the physicians. In addition, doctors were satisfied because a complete health examination was done.

*Reasons for Dissatisfaction*

As given in the above data, out of the 96 respondents who consulted some specialist for treatment, 16 respondents were found to be dissatisfied with treatment given by specialist. After identifying the reasons for satisfaction with the treatment, next question was to look in to the reasons for dissatisfaction for the respondents. So, question was asked about the reasons for dissatisfaction.

**Table 6.8 Distribution of Respondents on Basis of Reasons for**

**Dissatisfaction with the Treatment by the Physician**

| Most Important Reason Cited for Dissatisfaction | Number | Percentage |
|---|---|---|
| Diagnosis was not done properly | 6 | 37.50% |
| Treatment was not satisfactory | 2 | 12.50% |
| Behavior of physician was casual | 3 | 18.75% |
| Treatment details were not kept confidential | 5 | 31.25% |
| Total | 16 | 100% |

Table 6.8 explains that out of total 16 respondents who were asked to tell about the most important reason for their dissatisfaction from the physician, 6 (37.50%)

respondents answered that their diagnosis was not done properly by the physician. Other 5 (31.25%) respondents stated that the treatment details were not kept confidential. However, 3 (18.75%) respondents revealed that their illness was not taken seriously, while 2 (12.50%) respondents said that the treatment was not satisfactory.

Above findings demonstrated the various reasons for dissatisfaction with the treatment. Similarly, in Case 014, the 'doctor-patient' was dissatisfied with the treatment because his eye problem was not diagnosed properly by the doctor and later on his problem got aggravated.

In the above section, experiences of 'doctor as patient' had been discussed. However, we have to take into account the experiences which doctors had while treating 'doctor-patients' who were equally educated professionally. So, in the next section, experiences of the physician treating a 'doctor-patient' have been discussed.

## EXPERIENCES OF 'PHYSICIAN' OF 'DOCTOR-PATIENT'

A physician may also have different types of experiences during the treatment of a 'doctor-patient'. These experiences can be recognized by getting information regarding the opportunity of treating 'doctor-patients' by the physicians and afterwards analyzing the perception of physician about treating 'doctor-patient'.

### Experience of Treating 'Doctor-Patients'

To know about the experiences of physicians while treating the 'doctor-patients', the first question arises whether being physicians they have ever treated 'doctor-patients'. So, the question was asked in this regard from all the 240 respondents.

**Table 6.9 Distribution of Respondents on the Basis of experience of Treating a 'Doctor-Patient'**

| City | Experience of Treating a 'Doctor-patient' | | Total |
| --- | --- | --- | --- |
| | Yes | No | |
| Patiala | 79 (79.00%) | 21 (21.00%) | 100 (41.67%) |
| Amritsar | 120 (85.71%) | 20 (14.28%) | 140 (58.33%) |
| Total | 199 (82.91%) | 41 (17.08%) | 240 (100%) |

Table 6.9 indicates that out of 240 respondents, 199 (82.91%) had treated the 'doctor-patient' one or the other time in their practice period whereas 41 (17.08%) respondents had never treated a doctor as patient.

As mentioned in chapter II, 41 respondents were teaching in medical college, so they were not in practice of treating patients. So in this section, majority i.e. 199 (82.91%) doctors had got the opportunity of treating a 'doctor-patient' at least once in their career.

Also, during Focused Group Discussion all the doctors said that they had treated a 'doctor-patient' in their medical practice except for one doctor who was child specialist.

**Perception about Behaviour of 'Doctor-Patient'**

The perception of the physician about the behaviour of the 'doctor-patient' can be judged by knowing the perception of physician about the treating the 'doctor-patient', compliance of 'doctor-patient' with the advice of physician and regularity of follow-ups during treatment.

***Perception about Treatment of 'Doctor-Patient'***

Is treating the health related problem of a doctor is different from treating the illness of a common man? To get the answer of this question, the researcher asked question from physicians to know about their perception about whether doctors as patients are difficult or easy to treat or their behavior is same as that of routine patients.

**Table 6.10 Distribution of Respondents' Perception about Treating 'Doctor-Patient'**

| Treatment of 'Doctor-Patient' | Patiala | Amritsar | Total |
|---|---|---|---|
| Easy to treat | 7 (8.86%) | 17 (14.17%) | 24 (12.06%) |
| Difficult to treat | 60 (75.94%) | 91 (75.83%) | 151 (75.87%) |
| Same as normal patients | 12 (15.18%) | 12 (10.00%) | 24 (12.06%) |
| Total | 79 (39.69%) | 120 (60.30%) | 199 (100%) |

Data in the Table 6.10 show that 151 (75.87%) respondents out of total 199 respondents said that it is difficult to treat the 'doctor-patient' , 24 (12.06%)

respondents felt that 'doctor-patients' were easy to treat, and rest 24 (12.06%) respondents told that treating 'doctor-patient' was like routine patient. Thus from the data it seems that majority of respondents i.e. 151 (75.87%) perceived that 'doctor-patients' were difficult to treat.

During Focused Group Discussion, most of the participants told that doctors as patients were difficult to treat whereas few doctors, for instance, Dr. F and Dr. C said that treating a 'doctor-patient' was a pleasant experience.

### Perception about Compliance with Doctor's Advice

Compliance with doctor*'s* advice can be determined by the extent to which a patient shows adherence to taking medicines and changing lifestyle in consonance with advice of doctor. During the treatment it is important that patient should abide by the doctor's advice for speedy recovery. Approximately forty percent patients suffering from chronic diseases do not take medication prescribed by the doctor (Lee, Grace & Taylor, 2006). There will be a greater impact on the health of the people if there is an increase in compliance with medical advice rather than making improvement in medical treatment (WHO, 2003). So, better health outcomes depend upon the extent of compliance with the medical advice.

Therefore, in our research, we wanted to find out whether doctors as patients abide by doctor's advice so as to determine the sincerity to recover from illness. Question was asked from the doctors treating a 'doctor-patients' about compliance of their patients with their advice.

**Table 6.11 Distribution of Respondents' Perception about Compliance with**

**Doctor's Advice**

| City | Compliance with Doctor's Advice | | | Total |
|---|---|---|---|---|
| | Not at all | Occasionally | Always | |
| Patiala | 2 (2.53%) | 43 (54.43%) | 34 (43.03%) | 79 (41.67%) |
| Amritsar | 10 (8.33%) | 64 (53.33%) | 46 (38.33%) | 120 (58.33%) |
| Total | 12 (6.03%) | 107 (53.76%) | 80 (40.20%) | 199 (100%) |

Table 6.11 depicts the response of physician of 'doctor-patients' about following the doctors' advice by their 'doctor-patients'. Out of total 199 respondents who had ever treated a 'doctor-patient', 107 (53.76%) respondents told that 'doctor-patients' 'occasionally' observed the doctors' advice, 80 (40.20%) felt that 'doctor-patients' 'always' abide by advice and 12 (6.03%) respondents said that 'doctor-patients' 'not at all' showed compliance with the doctors' advice.

Thus maximum respondents (53.76%) 'occasionally' followed the doctor's advice that showed the callous attitude of 'doctor-patients' as far as their treatment was concerned. However, there was significant number (40.20%) of 'doctor-patients' who always showed observance to doctors' advice.

### *Perception about Follow Ups/ Regular Check-ups by 'Doctor-Patient'*

During the course of treatment, regular visit of patient to doctor is very necessary not only to make out the progress in recovery from disease but also to early detect the complications due to chronic disease. Frequency of medical examination may increase in an ailing condition that requires continuous care.

As already said that doctors show negligence and callousness in their treatment, so question was asked from physician who had ever treated a 'doctor-patient' to know that whether doctors as patients come up for follow-ups or regular check-ups during course of treatment.

**Table 6.12 Distribution of Respondents' Perception about Follow-ups/ Regular Check-ups by 'Doctor-Patient'**

| City | Follow-ups/ Regular Check-ups by 'Doctor-Patient' | | | Total |
|------|-----------|--------------|--------|-------|
|      | Not at all | Occasionally | Mostly |       |
| Patiala | 14 (17.72%) | 44 (55.69%) | 21(26.58%) | 79 (41.67%) |
| Amritsar | 17 (14.16%) | 64 (53.33%) | 39 (32.50%) | 120 (58.33%) |
| Total | 31 (15.57%) | 108 (54.27%) | 60 (30.15%) | 199 (100%) |

As shown in the above table 6.12, out of 199 respondents, 108 (54.27%) respondents felt that 'doctor-patients' 'occasionally' came for follow-ups, 60 (30.15%)

respondents' response was 'mostly' and 31 (15.57%) respondents gave the response 'not at all' when asked about the follow-ups routine of 'doctor-patients' during treatment.

The data show that according to most (69.84%) of the respondents, 'doctor-patients' did not follow regular health check-ups. There were only 60 (30.15%) respondents who were of the views that 'doctor-patient' come for the follow-ups 'mostly'. Here again 'doctor-patients' insensitive attitude about their chronic illness comes forth as they were not coming for regular health check-ups.

During Focused Group Discussion, reasons for difficulty in treating 'doctor-patients' were discussed. One of the participants i.e. Dr. A was of the opinion that 'doctor-patients' were always very much inquisitive and anxious about their health related issues. Whereas Dr. L mentioned that 'doctor-patients' conceal their unhealthy habits. Another participant, Dr. I, told that 'doctor-patients' do not show compliance with the doctor's advice.

II

## COPING MECHANISM

Compas et al. (2001) gave the definition of coping as, "conscious and volitional efforts to regulate emotion, cognition, behavior, physiology, and the environment in response to stressful events or circumstances (p.89)" (as cited in Compas, Jaser, Dunn & Rodriguez, 2012). Any kind of health related problem especially chronic illness brings with it a number of difficult situations such as chronic pain, interference with physical and social functioning, emotional trauma, prolonged and complex medical treatment etc. These difficult situations need adjustments at the physical as well as at the emotional level. So, coping mechanism plays an important role in readjustment of the ailing person in the society.

According to Compas et al. (2012) coping mechanism is based upon "a control-based model" and involves different types of strategies i.e. active coping or primary control, accommodative coping or secondary control and passive coping or disengagement. In active coping, primary effort is to manage one's feelings and to have a control over cause of stress. Accommodative coping or secondary control is associated with the efforts to adjust with cause of stress whereas passive coping or disengagement includes efforts to evade or refute the stressor. Accommodative coping or secondary control plays an important role in the successful adjustment of people to chronic illnesses whereas disengagement or passive shows poor adjustments. Primary control or active coping has mixed results (Compas et al., 2012).

Thus, a person suffering from lifestyle related disease may adopt various strategies to manage the chronic health condition. These strategies are taking medicines and precautions, undergoing regular health check-ups, changing lifestyle, doing yoga, engage in leisure activities etc. to de-stress oneself. Doctors are assumed to cope better with all the health related issues as compared to normal human beings. It was, therefore, desired to know whether or not the respondents had developed some mechanisms to cope up with the lifestyle related diseases. Thus, questions were asked from the unhealthy respondents about different ways that can be adopted to manage the chronic diseases.

**Medical Treatment as Coping Mechanism**

When a person develops any kind of chronic health condition or illness, first and foremost inclination of every person is to seek medical advice. The medical advice involves intake of medicines regularly. As stated earlier, in chronic illness adherence to medicines intake is poor.

So, researcher was interested in asking questions about regularity in taking medicines, form of medicine used and frequency of taking medicine by the respondents.

***Regularity in Taking Medicine for Chronic Illness***

After the detection of a disease, it is essential to take a proper treatment for the disease so that it remains in control and additional damage to the body can be avoided. Proper treatment includes regular intake of medicine for high blood pressure, high blood sugar level and for any other chronic illness. Irregular intake of medicine may not cure the diseased conditions and may result further aggravation of illness. Question was asked from the 130 unhealthy respondents regarding regularity in taking medicine.

**Table 6.13 Distribution of Respondents on the Basis of Regularity in**

**Taking Medicine per Day**

| Disease | Regularity in Taking Medicine | | Total* |
|---|---|---|---|
| | **Irregular** | **Regular** | |
| Blood Pressure | 19 (26.01%) | 54 (73.97%) | 73 (56.15%) |
| Blood Sugar | 6 (17.64%) | 28 (82.35%) | 34 (26.15%) |
| Other Diseases (Arthritis, Respiratory Disease, Spondylitis, Thyroid etc.) | 20 (30.79%) | 45 (69.23%) | 65 (50.00%) |

*Multiple Responses

Data shown in the Table 6.13 specify that 19 (26.01%) respondents were irregular in taking medicine whereas 54 (73.97%) respondents regularly took medicine for high blood pressure. As already said, there were 34 respondents suffering from diabetes and out of these 34 diabetic respondents, 28 (82.35%) were regular and 6 (17.64%) were irregular in taking medicine.

Out of total 65 respondents in case of the other chronic conditions like arthritis, respiratory problems, thyroid etc., 45 (69.23%) respondents took medicine regularly, 20 (30.79%) respondents were irregular in taking medicine.

Data in the above table indicate that majority of the respondents were regular in taking medicine in their respective chronic illnesses i.e. high blood pressure, high blood sugar and other chronic conditions. However, there is also small number (45) of respondents who were not taking medicines regularly.

In most of the case studies, regular intake of medicine by 'doctor-patients' was observed.

***Form of Medicine***

Generally two forms of medicine are used for treatment. One form is Allopathy system of medicine which is widely used globally and the other form of medicine is traditional medicine also known as alternative form of medicine. Alternative form of medicine practiced in India includes Ayurvedic, Homeopathic, Unani, Naturopathy etc.

While exploring the treatment taken for the lifestyle related diseases, we wanted to know about the trust of Allopathic doctors in different systems of medicine. So, question was asked from the respondents about the same.

**Table 6.14 Distribution of Respondents on the Basis of**

**Trust in the Form of Medicine**

| City | Trust in the Form of Medicine | | | Total |
|---|---|---|---|---|
| | **Ayurveda** | **Homeopathy** | **Allopathy** | |
| Patiala | 4 (7.27%) | 12 (21.81%) | 39 (70.90%) | 55 (41.67%) |
| Amritsar | 8 (10.67%) | 5 (6.67%) | 62 (82.67%) | 75 (58.33%) |
| Total | 12 (9.23%) | 17 (13.07%) | 101 (77.69%) | 130 (100%) |

Table 6.14 indicates that 101 (77.69%) respondents trusted in Allopathy that means they did not believe in any alternative form of medicine, only 17 (13.07%) believed in homeopathy and rest 12 (9.23%) trusted Ayurvedic medicine for their treatment.

Thus, majority (77.69%) of respondents believed in Allopathy medicine for their treatment. This may be due to the fact that our sample dealt with doctors practicing Allopathy. Their belief is more in their form of medicine than other forms of medicine.

**Coping Up by Taking Precautions**

Due to the development of lifestyle related diseases, a person has to take a lot of precautions along with regular intake of medicine. This may include restriction on intake of particular components in diet e.g. salt for hypertension and sugar for diabetes. So, taking precautions are essential to deal with the diseased condition efficiently. It was desired by the researcher to know about coping up with the disease by taking precautions among respondents.

Table 6.15 Distribution of Respondents' Perception of<br>Coping Up by Taking Precautions

| City | Coping up by Taking Precautions | | | Total |
|---|---|---|---|---|
| | **Not at all** | **Sometimes** | **Mostly** | |
| Patiala | 0 (0.00%) | 22 (40.00%) | 33 (60.00%) | 55 (42.30%) |
| Amritsar | 1 (1.33%) | 39 (52.00%) | 35 (46.67%) | 75 (57.69%) |
| Total | 1 (0.76%) | 61 (46.92%) | 68 (52.30%) | 130 (100%) |

Table 6.15 mentions that out of 130 unhealthy respondents, 35 (46.67%) respondents from Amritsar and 33 (60%) respondents from Patiala i.e. 68 (52.30%) respondents coped up with their illness by taking precautions 'mostly'. There were 61 (46.92%) respondents i.e. 39 (52%) from Amritsar and 22 (40%) from Patiala who coped up by taking precautions 'sometimes' whereas only 1 (0.76%) unhealthy respondent from both the cities 'not at all' coped up with the ailing condition by taking precautions.

The data show that most of the unhealthy respondents (99%) managed their chronic diseased condition by taking precautions either 'sometimes' or 'mostly'.

**Coping With the Help of Regular Health Check-ups**

Regular health checkups are indispensible for the routine health update and early detection of the health related problem. Normally, doctors instruct all the people whether suffering from some health trouble or not to go for regular health check-ups at regular interval of time. So, researcher was interested in detecting the presence of undergoing the regular health check-ups among doctors suffering from chronic illness. Question was asked about presence of routine health check-ups from unhealthy respondents.

Table 6.16 Distribution of Respondents on the Basis of Regularity of<br>Routine Health Check-ups in a Year

| City | Regularity of Routine Health Check-ups | | Total |
|---|---|---|---|
| | **Irregular** | **Regular** | |
| Patiala | 12 (21.81%) | 43 (78.18%) | 55 (42.30%) |
| Amritsar | 15 (20.00%) | 60 (80.00%) | 75 (57.69%) |
| Total | 27 (20.76%) | 103 (79.23%) | 130 (100%) |

Table 6.16 depicts that out of total 130 unhealthy respondents, 27 (20.76%) respondents were irregular whereas 103 (79.23%) were regular in their health check-ups. Thus, majority (79.23%) of unhealthy respondents went for regular health check-ups.

Irregularity of health checkups has also been observed in Case Study 003 where even after suffering from hypertension at the young age of 24, the patient was not undergoing regular medical checkups.

### *Frequency of Regular Health Check-ups*

As said earlier, 27 (20.76%) respondents were irregular and 103 (79.23%) were regular in their health check-ups. Now, next question arises that those who were regular in health check-ups, for how many times in a year they go for check-ups. This way we can know the awareness of respondents about their health needs.

**Table 6.17 Distribution of Respondents on the Basis of Frequency of**

**Regular Health Check-ups**

| City | Frequency of Regular Health Check-ups | | | Total |
|---|---|---|---|---|
| | Once a year | 2-3 times a year | >3 times a year | |
| Patiala | 22 (51.16%) | 15 (34.88%) | 6 (13.95%) | 43 (41.74%) |
| Amritsar | 33 (55.00%) | 19 (31.67%) | 8 (13.33%) | 60 (58.25%) |
| Total | 55 (53.39%) | 34 (33.00%) | 14 (13.59%) | 103 (100%) |

As shown in the Table 6.17, out of 103 respondents having regular health check-ups, 55 (53.39%) respondents said that they went for health check-ups once a year, 34 (33%) respondents told that they usually went for routine health check-ups for 2-3 times in one year. Other 14 (13.59%) respondents underwent medical check-ups more than three times a year.

Data show that maximum numbers (55) of respondents were undergoing routine medical check-ups once a year whereas significant numbers (48) of respondents went for medical check-ups more than once in a year.

**Coping Up by Changing Lifestyle**

'Lifestyle' involves the attitudes, opinions, interests, and behaviors of an individual, a group and a culture. Since the lifestyle related diseases are mostly caused by faulty lifestyle, therefore to make changes in the lifestyle is imperative for the healthy living of a person as well as to manage the chronic condition.

However, it is difficult for all to change the lifestyle due to their social, psychological and practical conditions. Murray, Craig, Honey & House (2012) mentioned the social (family and friends support), psychological (beliefs and emotions) and practical factors (transport and other costs) influence the change in lifestyle behaviour and its maintenance. As to manage the lifestyle related disease is a continuous process, so, a person has to be persistent in his efforts to make lifestyle changes. The question was, thus, asked from the respondents to look in to their efforts in bringing the required changes in their lifestyle.

**Table 6.18 Distribution of Respondents' Perception of**

**Coping Up by Changing Lifestyle**

| City | Coping Up by Changing Lifestyle | | | Total |
|---|---|---|---|---|
| | **Not at all** | **Sometimes** | **Mostly** | |
| Patiala | 0 (0.00%) | 21 (38.18%) | 34 (61.81%) | 55 (42.30%) |
| Amritsar | 1 (1.33%) | 38 (50.67%) | 36 (48.00%) | 75 (57.69%) |
| Total | 1 (0.76%) | 59 (45.38%) | 70 (53.84%) | 130 (100%) |

Table 6.18 shows that out of 70 (53.84%) unhealthy respondents, 36 (48%) unhealthy respondents from Amritsar and 34 (61.81%) unhealthy respondents from Patiala changed their lifestyle to cope up with the illness 'mostly', other 59 (45.38%) unhealthy respondents i.e. 38 (50.67%) from Amritsar and 21 (38.18%) from Patiala changed their lifestyle 'sometimes' and 1 (0.76%) respondent from Amritsar did not change the lifestyle to cope up with the chronic disease.

The data depict that all the unhealthy respondents i.e. 129 respondents except 01 asserted that they had coped up with the disease by changing their lifestyle.

Some people may not be able to change their lifestyle even being aware of the harmful effects of unhealthy lifestyle. In case study 009, the doctor suffering from cardiac problem was following an unhealthy lifestyle even after the onset of the disease.

In the Focused Group Discussion, majority of the unhealthy participants stressed that change in lifestyle is mandatory for recovery. Some of the participants suggested for the lifestyle changes along with medication.

**Coping Up With the Help of Practice of Yoga**

Yoga is originated from Sanskrit word "Yuj" that means "to yoke or joint together". It includes exercise, stretching, aerobic exercise and meditation. It helps in integrating the mind and body by deep breathing, stretching, balanced posture and relaxation.

It is commonly believed that stress aggravates all the types of health related problems and also results in onset of chronic health conditions. Malathi and Damodaran (1999) discussed the positive role played by yoga in relieving stress. They argued that yoga not only helps in changing a person's attitude and response towards stress but also helps in increasing a feeling of wellbeing, relaxation, and self-confidence. As the stress reliever, role of yoga is considered important for coping up with the ailing condition.

Also, Eda (2014) reviewed a number of studies on beneficial effects of yoga on chronic conditions such as COPD and cancer and asserted that yoga might help the patients with chronic conditions by decreasing distress.

So, researcher wanted to know the inclination of unhealthy respondents towards practicing yoga to relieve stress due to chronic illness.

**Table 6.19 Distribution of Respondents on the Basis of
Coping Up with the Practice of Yoga**

| City | Practice of Yoga | | Total |
|---|---|---|---|
| | **Yes** | **No** | |
| Patiala | 21 (38.18%) | 34 (61.81%) | 55 (42.30%) |
| Amritsar | 33 (44.00%) | 42 (56.00%) | 75 (57.69%) |
| Total | 54 (41.53%) | 76 (58.46%) | 130 (100%) |

Table 6.19 depicts that out of 130 unhealthy respondents, 54 (41.53%) respondents were doing yoga and 76 (58.46%) respondents were not doing yoga to relieve the stress in order to cope up with ailing condition.

Out of 54 respondents, who were doing yoga, 21 (38.18%) belonged to Patiala and 33 (44%) were from Amritsar. Out of 76 respondents, who were not doing yoga, 34 (61.81%) and 42 (56%) were from Patiala and Amritsar respectively.

The data show that most (58.46%) of the respondents were not doing yoga. However 54 (41.53%) respondents were doing yoga to manage stress due to their diseased condition. The lack of yoga exercise may be due to the hectic lifestyle where doctors don't find time for doing such exercises.

In Case 012, the doctor said that he has been practicing yoga in the morning for last 20 years and he has no chronic illness. During Focused Group Discussion, one of the participants Dr. E suffering from asthma practiced yoga and meditation to get relief in ailing condition.

**Coping Up With the Help of Leisure Activities**

Leisure activities may not only facilitate the physical and mental healing of people but also acts as a stress reliever in chronic health conditions. Pressman et al. (2009) explored the role of leisure activities among people in recovering from stress and restoring physical and social resources. Importance of leisure activities in physical and social wellbeing of individuals was also discussed by Coleman & Iso-Ahola (1993). According to him, leisure time activities with the other people help in establishing social support network as well as acts as mediator in stress and healthy relationship (Coleman & Iso-Ahola, 1993).

As already said that long term stress results in to instigating physical health issues, so, it was desired to identify the types of leisure activities preferred by the 130 unhealthy respondents to relieve themselves from stress.

**Table 6.20 Distribution of Respondents on the Basis of**

**Coping Up with the Help of Leisure Activities**

| Performance of Leisure Activities | Patiala | Amritsar | Total* |
|---|---|---|---|
| Spending time with family | 4/55 | 11/75 | 15 (11.53%) |
| Spending time with friends and relatives | 10/55 | 10/75 | 20 (15.38%) |
| Watching T.V | 34/55 | 45/75 | 79 (60.76%) |
| Reading books | 21/55 | 34/75 | 55 (42.30%) |
| Other activities (listening to music, cooking, Dancing, gardening etc.) | 16/55 | 12/75 | 28 (21.53%) |
| No  time for leisure activities | 5/55 | 5/75 | 10 (7.69%) |

* Multiple Responses

As shown in Table 6.20, unhealthy respondents were involved in various leisure activities to relieve themselves from stress because of chronic conditions. These leisure activities were watching T.V (60.76%), reading books (42.30%), involving in other activities such as dancing, cooking and gardening etc. (21.53%), socializing with people (15.38%), and spending time with family (11.53%). However, 10 (7.69%) respondents out of total 130 unhealthy respondents also said that they did not engage in any leisure activity.

The most commonly (60.76%) performed leisure activity was watching T.V. and least commonly (11.53%) preferred was spending time with the family.

**Role of Family and Friends in Coping**

Informal networks such as family and friends not only provide the care giving services and useful information related to health care but also act as a psychological support during physical and mental distress ( Umberson, 1987).

Family and friends constitute the social support system for an individual. Social support also plays an important role in observing of positive and negative health behaviors related to exercise, eating, drinking or smoking etc. These behaviors may directly or indirectly influence the morbidity and mortality.

Further, every crisis in one's life is dealt with the support of family and friends. They help in managing the critical situation. Development of lifestyle related disease is also a time of crisis when the support of family and friends is needed to come out of that situation. So, question was asked from the respondents that to what extent the family and friends were helpful in coping up with the disease.

**Table 6.21 Distribution of Respondents' Perception of the Extent of Help from**

**Family and Social Ties in Coping with the Diseases**

| City | Extent of Help of Family and Social Ties in Coping with the Diseases | | | Total |
|------|------------|-----------|--------|-------|
| | **Not at all** | **Sometimes** | **Mostly** | |
| Patiala | 1 (1.81%) | 19 (34.54%) | 35 (63.63%) | 55 (42.30%) |
| Amritsar | 2 (2.67%) | 36 (48.00%) | 37 (49.33%) | 75 (57.69%) |
| Total | 3 (2.30%) | 55 (42.30%) | 72 (55.38%) | 130 (100%) |

Table 6.21 specifies that out of total 130 unhealthy respondents, 72 (55.38%) respondents said that family and social ties helped in coping up with the disease 'mostly', 55 (42.30%) respondents felt that family and social ties helped 'sometimes' and 3 (2.30%) respondents told that family and social ties 'not at all' helped in coping up with diseased condition.

Majority i.e. 127 (98%) of unhealthy respondents coped up more or less with the help of family and social ties.

During Focused Group Discussion, it was general perception that family and friends are proved to be their lifelines in the time of crisis during ailments. Without this support system, it would not be possible for them to come out of critical situation.

**SUMMARY**

In the first part of this chapter, experiences of doctors as patients and that of physician of 'doctor-patients' were discussed. In the second part, different coping strategies executed by the doctors as patients for recovering from diseased condition were observed.

On the basis of the data, it can easily be chalked out that a large number of 'doctor-patients' (60%) took their illness normally while on the other hand, a good number (40%) had the feeling of shock (34.61%), apprehension (46.15%) or depression (19.23%),. So, most common feeling was of apprehension for the future health and least common was that of depression.

Majority of the 'doctor-patients' (73.84%) preferred to consult some professional practitioner instead of practicing self-medication (26.15%). Most (52.08%) of the 'doctor-patients' did not want to go to familiar physicians for treatment because of fear of loss of confidentiality. Among familiar doctors, colleagues were preferred (60.86%) as compared to friends (32.60%) and relatives (6.52%) for taking treatment.

Majority (83.33%) of the 'doctor-patients' were satisfied with the treatment of their physician although there were few respondents (16.67%) who were not satisfied. The most common reason for satisfaction (27.50%) with the behavior of physician was the seriousness with which the ailing condition was dealt with whereas the most common reason for dissatisfaction (37.50%) was improper diagnosis.

Further, when we looked at the experiences of physician of 'doctor-patient', we found that physicians perceived that 'doctor-patients' were mostly difficult to treat (75.87%) because they show non-compliance (6.03%) or occasional compliance (53.76%) with doctor's advice and were negligent about the routine follow-ups (69.84%). This perception of physician about 'doctor-patient' is in consonance with the popular saying that 'doctors make bad patients'.

The coping up with diseased condition involved different coping strategies. The doctors as patients coped up with the help of taking medicine. The most preferred form of medicine was Allopathy (77.69%) rather than Homeopathy (13.07%) or Ayurvedic (9.23%). Regular intake of medicine was observed among doctors mostly but a small number (20.76%) of doctors were found to be irregular in their medicine intake. There were 52.30% 'doctor-patients' who took precautions on regular basis to cope up with the ailing condition. 'Doctor-patients' also coped up with the help of regular health check-ups (79.23%), changing the lifestyle mostly (53.84%), and with the help of practicing yoga (41.53%).

However, to reduce the stress due to illness different types of leisure activities were also performed by the respondents. The most preferred leisure activities were watching television (60.76%) and reading books (42.30%). Help of family and social ties during the time of crisis also facilitated a lot in coping with the lifestyle related diseases. More than half (55.38%) of the respondents coped up with the ailing condition with the help of family ties and friends 'mostly' and 42.30% respondents felt so 'sometimes' .

Hence, this chapter highlighted the experiences of doctors as patients and physicians of 'doctor-patients' in their respective statuses and also coping mechanism adopted by the 'doctor-patients' to manage the diseased condition.

# CHAPTER VII

# CASE STUDIES AND FOCUSED GROUP DISCUSSION

In the previous chapters, we have dealt with the quantitative data. It is imperative, however, to get qualitative information related to the objectives of the study for the deeper insight in to the subject. Thus, researcher tried to understand qualitative aspects of the problem under study with the help of Case Studies and Focused Group Discussion.

In this chapter, a detail description of Case Studies and Focused Group Discussion has been carried on. In total, seventeen (17) Case Studies and one (1) Focused Group Discussion were conducted for the better understanding of the issue.

In the first part of the chapter, Case Studies have been described and in the second part, Focused Group Discussion has been discussed.

## CASE STUDIES

According to Young (1956), "Case study is a method of exploring and analyzing the life of a social unit, be that a person, a family, institution, culture, group or even entire community." Case study is a comprehensive and intensive study of a social unit where all the aspects of a social unit are studied.

In the present study, the researcher selected some peculiar cases and tried to explore the different aspects of these cases with or without lifestyle related diseases. Further, the researcher    classified all these cases in different categories according to different reasons responsible for occurrence of lifestyle related diseases. Names have been changed in order to keep the confidentiality of the cases.

In some cases there was no family history of disease but still the respondents were reported with the chronic illness and in some other cases even after having a family history of various diseases, the respondents were leading a healthy life due to healthy lifestyle. In addition to this, role of lack of cial and emotional support system in causing diseases, negligence by the physician while treating the 'doctor-patient' and difficulty faced in coping mechanism have also been explored through some case studies.

**Unhealthy Lifestyle Leading to Diseases among Doctors (With a Family History)**

In following Case Studies family history of one or the other disease is there and an unhealthy lifestyle acted as catalyst for the occurrence of lifestyle related disease.

**Case: 001**

*Lack of exercise, sedentary lifestyle, stress, smoking and drinking habits and leading to Diabetes, Cardiac Problem and Hypertension.*

*Family history of disease: Heart disease and Diabetes*

Dr. Jatinder is 63 years old married male living in a nuclear family and working in Pharmacology department of a government hospital. He has been in this profession for more than 36 years and had a number of health issues. He has been suffering from diabetes for the last 12 years. Diabetes was detected when symptoms appeared like non-healing of fungal infection for a long time. Overtime he developed heart disease due to high blood glucose level and suffered a silent heart attack without warning 9 years ago. He also developed problem of hypertension 5 months ago which he think is due to stress of his chronic conditions.

The main reason for the development of all these health related problems is an unhealthy lifestyle along with the family history. According to respondent, he follows unhealthy lifestyle. He started smoking in his college for fun and did not realize that he has become addicted to smoking. He used to smoke minimum 12 cigarettes daily. He used to consume alcohol 4 days or more per week having 3-4 drinks at one time. Due to influence of his wife and adult children he quitted alcohol in 2008. He had not been able to quit smoking completely but had reduced the number of cigarettes. Though he had made few changes in his food habits after he came to know about his health issues but he was not involved in any regular physical activity. He has a sedentary lifestyle and always prefers lift over stairs.

His normal social activities, recreational activities, household activities, outdoor activities and eating habits suppress a lot due his chronic diseases. According to him, people avoid interaction with diseased person. He is not discouraged and worried because of his health related problems but he is more or less fearful and frustrated due to these problems. He went through physical and mental fatigue due to this. Coping up with the physical discomfort and fatigue was a challenge for him but psychologically he coped up with all the health issues very confidentially.

 The above case study depicts that unhealthy lifestyle which involved excessive use of alcohol and tobacco products, physical inactivity etc. along with family history played an important role for the causation of disease. Also, the respondent was not having the habit of regular medical check-ups. He came to know about the diseases only after the appearance of symptoms.

**Case: 002**

*Irregular and unhealthy diet pattern, physical inactivity, anxiety, habit of smoking and alcohol consumption led to Hypertension at a very young age of 18 years*

*Family History of disease: Hypertension (Parents), Diabetes (Father)*

Dr. Mohan is 56 years old married male living in nuclear family and working as Psychiatrist in government institution. He was detected with hypertension at a very young age of 18 years when he started preparation for medical entrance to secure admission into M.B.B.S.

He holds unhealthy lifestyle as well as anxiety responsible for hypertension at the age of 18 years and is taking treatment for hypertension for the more than 35 years. He was worried almost every day about lot of things like homework, tests, social life with friends etc. He did not want to make any mistakes in his studies especially his medical entrance tests.

During this period, anxiety induced stress had led him to follow an unhealthy lifestyle in addition to an irregular diet pattern and poor exercise routine. He relied on junk food mostly like chips, aerated drinks, French fries etc. He picked up smoking and drinking habits due to his peer pressure. Apart from this, he likes to read books, watching television and listening to music and all these activities are sedentary in nature. He is obese and follows a sedentary lifestyle which increases his exposure to various lifestyle diseases. He also survived a heart attack which forced him to quit smoking, alcohol, and follow a regular fitness routine along with regular health check-ups which is helping him in regaining his physical fitness and increase his lifespan.

He has a family history of hypertension and diabetes and he is suffering from the same and has already survived a heart attack at a very young age. He says such problems are common after age of 50 years but it came as a shock to him that he is suffering from hypertension at such a young age. Despite that he is leading a normal social life but mentally he lives with the feeling of discouragement, fearfulness.

Thus, above case study shows that unhealthy lifestyle can be a reason for an illness at a very young age and if required precautions are not taken at the initial level then it may lead to a critical condition. It is evident in this case study that failure on the part of respondent to take required precautions led to a major lifestyle related disease. Also, psychological impact of the chronic illness has been observed just like a common man.

**Case: 003**

*Lack of exercise and unhealthy diet lead to Hypertension at a young age of 24 years*

*Family History of disease: Hypertension (Parents)*

Dr. Jatin is 31 years old child specialist in private practice. He is in practice for last two years. He is suffering from hypertension for the last 7 years and has been taking anti-hypertensive medicine for seven years. According to him, unhealthy diet and lack of exercise are major reasons for his health related problem. Both of his parents are also suffering from hypertension.

As far as the prevalence of risk factors are concerned, his daily eating schedule is irregular due to his carelessness. He is fond of processed meat products and has a habit of regularly eating food in food joints and restaurants. He is also not taking the recommended quantity of fruits, vegetables or legumes and dairy products.

Due to lack of time, he is not very much regular in physical workout. He considers his work very stressful. He works for seven days in a week and more than eight hours a day. He says "There is no doubt that my work is very stressful and time demanding but I enjoy my work, no doubt, it is very difficult to squeeze out time for physical activity after attending patients back to back and handling emergency cases." He told that due to his work load he cannot even get 8 hours of sleep daily.

Though the chronic illness has negligible effect on his social activities but it has marked psychological effect. Sometimes a feeling of discouragement, fearfulness, worry and frustration come to him as a result of his health related issues. He has coped moderately well with the disease but he is not undergoing a routine medical check-ups. He is not a gregarious person and prefers reading books in free time. Therefore most of his day is sedentary and involves very less in physical activity.

Here, risk factors responsible for causation of hypertension are both modifiable and non-modifiable. Non-modifiable factors are genetics because both parents of respondent are hypertensive and modifiable factors are unhealthy lifestyle and lack of exercise, lack of sleep etc. The modifiable factors in this case acted as catalyst for the onset of hypertension at a young age of 24 years.

**Case: 004**

*Unhealthy diet, negligence, obesity and smoking lead to Hypertension and Cardiac problem*

*Family history of disease: Hypertension (Mother)*

Dr. Yogesh is 48 years old married male living in a nuclear family set up. He is in the government job for the last 22 years. He is suffering from hypertension for past 10 years and from cardiac problem for the last 7 years. Smoking and unhealthy lifestyle have been assigned as the main reasons for the development of problem.

He has a family history of hypertension but no family history of cardiac problem. Even after knowing that his mother has problem of hypertension and he has more chances of having it he still continued with his unhealthy lifestyle and ignored symptoms like fatigue and continuous headache. His problem of high blood pressure put strain on his heart and he developed heart problem. Though he is regular in his eating schedule but he has a habit of eating outside and taking junk and fast food frequently. He goes to eat at restaurants 2-3 times a week and every now and then he orders home delivery from his favorite food joints.

Required consumption of fruits, vegetables and milk is missing in his diet and he is taking high quantity of caffeine products like tea and coffee. He used to smoke but left it 7 years ago after the cardiac problem. He is taking a controlled quantity of alcohol for the last 20 years. He says "I believe, you are what you eat. So after the appearance of cardiac problem, I tried to follow a healthy lifestyle and quitting smoking completely which was hardest for me." He is not doing any physical activity and he is overweight.

He felt depressed after knowing about his illness. He says, "When my doctor disclosed me my cardiac problem, it appeared to me that everything has ended." His social, recreational, household and outdoor activities are affected 'moderately' and his eating habits are affected the most due to chronic condition. He quite often feels discouragement, fearfulness, worry and frustration. He has a feeling of physical and mental fatigue sometimes and his efficiency of work is also affected. He used to work a lot in day but now after the cardiac problem he feels tired even after a little work.

He tried to cope up with his problem by taking medicine but at the practical level coping mechanism was difficult for him. He was not very much efficient in coping up with the changes in social and family ties, lifestyle etc. Confidence level to deal with the physical discomfort, mental or emotional distress and fatigue was also low.

Hence, from the above case study it is clear that unhealthy lifestyle like unhealthy diet, smoking and obesity can be the causative factors for the onset of a disease even when there is no family history of cardiac disease. Also, doctors too behave like a common man when suffering from disease. They are also socially and psychologically affected by the illness and they find it difficult to cope up with the changes in lifestyle.

**Case: 005**

*Physical inactivity, irregular and unhealthy diet pattern, sedentary lifestyle led to Hypothyroidism and Diabetes.*

*Family history of disease: Diabetes*

Dr. Rajesh is 40 years old married male living in joint family and is working in government hospital. He has been suffering from hypothyroidism for the last 12 years and diabetes for more than 4 years. His unhealthy lifestyle is the main reason for his chronic illnesses. He prefers eating foods with high sugar and high fat content. His daily breakfast comprises of prantha and tea. Due to this type of diet and physical inactivity he has a very unhealthy BMI. Moreover, he has an irregular eating schedule due to his busy schedule. Even though he should quit the products with sugar but he is unable to avoid sugar completely which he realizes is not good for his health. He is not involved in any kind of physical activity. His habit of unhealthy eating and no physical workout has made him obese.

Despite having a family history of diabetes, he was not regular in routine medical check-ups. He came to know about his illness when the symptoms appeared. After the detection of diabetes, he is trying to take a healthy and balanced diet. The respondent is not very much social but to deal with anxiety issues due to health related problem, he increased his social and recreational activities. He was very much affected psychologically by his disease. He tried to deal with physical fatigue and discomfort confidently but he was less confident to deal with the emotional distress caused by the disease.

So, this case study reveals that like a commoner the respondent underwent medical examination only after appearance of symptoms and coping mechanism took a long time. Hence, doctors do not do what they preach.

**Stressful Lifestyle Leading to Diseases among Doctors (Without a Family History)**

In this section, Case Studies without the family history of disease have been discussed. Here, stress has been assigned as the main reason for the occurrence of lifestyle related diseases. Importantly, all these Cases are not having a family history of diseases.

**Case: 006**

*Academic stress leading to Cardiac Problem at the young age of 28 years*

*Family History of disease: Negative*

Dr. Inderjeet is 49 years old Sikh married male working in a government hospital and is post-graduate in Pharmacology without any family history of cardiac problem. Being from a middle class nuclear family, he was under tremendous pressure to secure a seat in government medical college. Pressure of studies in medical college increased the stress level. He used to get very exhausted and hardly any time was left for other things. He developed irregular eating and sleeping schedule. Therefore his health was affected due to his unhealthy and sedentary lifestyle. After experiencing heart palpitations and chest pain he went to see a heart specialist in his own hospital. After going through various tests he was diagnosed with heart problem and he had to undergo a bypass surgery immediately at young age of 28 years. He found it difficult to absorb the reality of his illness. Though his disease did not interfere with his normal social, recreational and household activities but it has noticeable effect on his eating habits. He started eating more healthy home cooked food and kept himself on a low sodium and low fat diet.

His cardiac problem had a striking effect on his psychology. He usually feels fearful and worried by his chronic disease. Physical and mental fatigue is more frequent and most of the time he feels like taking a break from works to relieve him from stress. He couldn't manage his stress and was not able to take corrective action to come out of his stress.

This case study reveals that despite not having a family history of disease, the respondent is having cardiac problem. Stress and unhealthy lifestyle are the major threats for the development of a disease. Respondent began to follow a healthy lifestyle only after the appearance of disease. Like a common man he also had a feeling of shock, disbelief and depression on knowing about the problem. Also, psychological coping was quite difficult for him like a commoner.

**Case: 007**

*Stress due to frequent Job transfers lead to Hypertension*

*Family History of disease: Negative*

Dr. Maninder is 66 years old married male from an upper middle class family. He is a postgraduate in Pathology and at present running his own laboratory. Previously, he was in a government job from 1979 to 2005. He says that though he understand that transfers help employee gain a broader experience in work and are helpful in career but if the transfers are more frequent then they take toll on personal life. With every transfer he had to adjust to a new environment and new circumstances.

Moreover, hectic job conditions caused extreme tiredness and fatigue and he could not pursue any physical activity despite being good badminton player. Due to transfer at far off places he could not relocate his family with him everywhere as he did not want them to suffer. He realized that transfers in his job are unavoidable and he was stressed as he could not balance his personal and professional life. All the stress started interfering with his health too. Due to this continuous stress, he was detected with hypertension at an age of 40 years.

When he felt helpless in carrying on his professional and personal obligations, he took voluntary retirement. He opened a private pathology laboratory in his own city. In a private set up he is quite satisfied with his personal and professional life. Now he has less job stress and more time for his personal life. According to him, job stress due to frequent transfers is the reason for the development of hypertension.

The respondent has no family history of hypertension. Stress, physical inactivity and obesity had adverse effects on his health. He is not habitual exerciser and due to this he has put on the extra weight. Moreover, he wasn't careful about his health because despite detection of the disease, he started to take treatment quite late.

As a Pathologist he had a sedentary working environment which involves long hours of sitting and even his leisure time activities in home or otherwise are sedentary like watching television and reading books.

As far as the social, psychological and economic effects are concerned, the hypertension did not interfere with his normal social activities with family, friends and neighbors, household and outdoor activities but it interfered slightly with eating habits and recreational activities. He was slightly discouraged and fearful initially and had a feeling of physical and mental fatigue due to his illness. Social and psychological coping with the disease was quite easy for him afterwards.

Primarily job related stress is the main reason enlisted by the respondent for his chronic health condition but unhealthy lifestyle such as physical inactivity and obesity are the precipitating factors for the development of disease. In addition to this, he still does not have an active lifestyle.

No family history of disease reveals that genetic inheritance should not be considered as the sole reason for the development of a chronic disease.

**Case: 008**

*Stress during Post-graduation led to Hypertension and Chronic Kidney Disease.*

*Family History of disease: Negative*

Dr. Manoj is 53 years married male from upper middle class family. He is working as a specialist in Surgery in government hospital and has been suffering from hypertension and chronic kidney disease for the last fifteen and twelve years respectively. He never went for any health check-up and got to know about his kidney problems only on the onset of severe abdominal pain.

He has no history of hypertension and kidney related diseases in his family. According to him, stress during his post-graduation is one of the major reasons for his present health. According to him, he was brilliant in his academics and was a topper throughout his academic life. Medical study was very hectic and generated high levels of stress. Further, it got compounded with a sedentary lifestyle. He developed unhealthy eating habits. He also attributes his present condition to fewer intakes of fruits, vegetables or legumes and dairy products and more intakes of junk food and aerated drinks during his younger days. He had less physical activity due to this he became obese. He has been trying to lose weight for the past six months but hasn't succeeded despite bringing changes in his exercise schedule.

Though socially and economically, he isn't much affected by his health condition but the psychological impact of it is very high. He says "My life has gone out of control due to my kidney disease. Living with this disease is not easy." He is disheartened, scared and worried. He most of the times experiences mental and physical exertion because of his illness.

The above case study once again highlighted that even doctors ignore their health issues and delay diagnosis till the symptoms get aggravated. Moreover, the case also put light towards the hypothesis that family history is not the only causative factor for getting lifestyle related diseases.

**Case: 009**

*Stress due to workaholic attitude leading to Cardiac Problem*

*Family History of disease: Negative*

Dr. Yograj is 74 years old married male in private practice and lives in joint family. He developed cardiac problem 32 years ago at the age of 42. According to him, stress due to overwork was the main reason for the development of cardiac problem. In the initial years of his career he was a workaholic. He wanted to be one of the best in his field of expertise. He used to start his day early and see as many patients as possible. Moreover, fascination for his field made him pursue medical research which consumed a lot of his leisure time. Due to this excessive work load, he was not able to maintain a healthy lifestyle and ultimately developed heart problem. He was taken aback that he has developed the cardiac problem despite having no family history. He is teetotaler and non-smoker.

Even after the onset of heart problem he is following an unhealthy lifestyle. He is still not taking breaks in between his job hours. Though he has reduced consuming junk food but still he is not regular with his meals. Every now and then he skips his lunch.

Physical inactivity has made him overweight. He is obese and he is not in a position to do regular physical activity due to his health related problem and busy schedule. He is working seven days a week and his working hours depend upon the situation. Usually he is so tired after his work in the hospital that he fails to pursue any physical activity. But after the persuasion from his physician he tried to adopt an active lifestyle. Now, his life is moderately active and his leisure time activities are reading books and watching T.V. and brisk walking every day.

As far as the effects of cardiac problem are concerned, he is affected socially due to restricted recreational, outdoor and household activities. There is major effect on his eating habits. Psychological effect can be seen because of feelings of dissuasion, apprehension, anxiousness, mental fatigue and disturbance due to cardiac problem.

The respondent more or less coped with the changes in social and family ties and daily routine. He managed to cope up with the physical discomfort and emotional distress very confidently. Regular medicines intake help in coping up the cardiac problem.

**Case: 010**

*Early life professional stresses and unhealthy lifestyle lead to Rheumatoid Arthritis*

*Family History of disease: Negative*

Dr. Yamini is 45 years old married women from upper middle class family doing job in government hospital under Punjab Civil and Medical services (PCMS) for the last 15 years.

She says her both parents are living a healthy life even at age of 70 years. But she has been suffering from rheumatoid arthritis for the last ten years and is also having high levels of thyroid for last one and a half years. With no family history of such diseases, she holds stress, unhealthy diet and lack of exercise responsible for her illness.

During her house job period in government hospital, she used to have a very busy schedule. Due to this busy job, irregular shifts and her own carelessness she developed irregular diet pattern and started missing her meals. She did not spare time for herself and for her family. Moreover, lack of time for regular physical workout resulted into her present medical situation over a period of time. She feels that her job is complicated and carries a lot of responsibilities which over time has developed stress which lead to the development of rheumatoid arthritis at the young age of 35 years.

She admits that as a doctor she generally tells the patients to have routine medical check-ups but in her own case, she underwent medical examination only when the first symptoms appeared like pain and stiffness in joints. At first she ignored the problem because she thought it is because of tiredness but she felt shocked when she was diagnosed with rheumatoid arthritis.

Rheumatoid arthritis has a considerable effect on her social and psychological wellbeing. The disease has not only restricted her social activities with family and friends but it has also affected his personal and professional life. She became emotional while discussing her chronic health issues.

The above case study makes amply clear that development of lifestyle related diseases is not an overnight process and takes a long time to develop and an unhealthy lifestyle provides a mushrooming base for the same. Second, family history is not a sole reason for developing such diseases. A person with no family history can have a chronic illness due to his or her unhealthy lifestyle and stress in daily life plays a crucial role in aggravating the health related problem. Third, doctors are also human beings; they can also have a feeling of discouragement and find difficulty in coping up the disease.

**Healthy Lifestyle Results in Disease Free Life (Despite Family History of Diseases)**

This section deals with the cases where the respondents maintained a healthy lifestyle throughout their life and prevented the occurrence of lifestyle related diseases even with a family history of disease.

**Case: 011**

*Despite having a family history of Hypertension, Diabetes and Cardiac problem the respondent is healthy*

*Family History of disease: Hypertension and Diabetes (Mother), Cardiac Problem (Father)*

Dr. Gautum is 50 years married male working as a surgeon in a government hospital. He lives in nuclear family. His mother is 76 years old and is a patient of hypertension and diabetes and his father 80 years of age has cardiac problem. Despite having a family history of these diseases he is completely healthy even at the age of 50 years. The reason of his good health according to him is his active and healthy lifestyle.

He says, "Your health is your first wealth." He takes a special care of what he consumes. He has a regular eating schedule and has been taking healthy and balanced diet for more than 25 years. He avoids having processed food and prefers eating green vegetables and fruits. For snacks also he chooses foods like fruits, dry fruits, nuts etc. One aspect he emphasized is that he dines early in the evening and frequently does fasting. During the fasting days he avoids taking salt and eats only once in a day. He is regularly doing physical work out such as stretching and strengthening exercises, walking, bicycling and other aerobic exercises. He has been very active member of local bicycling club and loves playing Tennis. He is non-smoker and he never consumed alcohol. He stays away from processed foods with excess oil, sugar and salt. He is very social and prefers to interact with the people in his free time. Even during social gatherings he prefers eating healthy foods like green salad or curd.

He considers his job very sensitive and sometimes dangerous also as many times people engage in altercations with doctors and also resort to violence. He is against the Consumer Protection Act where doctors are sometimes falsely implicated by the patients.

As already mentioned, the respondent has family history of many diseases. Despite having a family history of diseases, the respondent is healthy. According to respondent, the credit goes to his healthy lifestyle. He says "we are brand ambassadors of good health and we should act as role models for people in society".

From the above case study, it is clear that the diseases like diabetes, hypertension and cardiac problem which were once considered as solely genetic are not completely genetic. Lifestyle of an individual is also a deciding factor for causation of disease. This is also revealed by World Health Organization that 80% of diabetes and hypertension and more than 40% of cancers are preventable by following a healthy lifestyle.

**Case: 012**

*Family history of Hypertension but respondents has no chronic disease.*

*Family History of disease: Hypertension*

Dr. Mohinder is 62 years old male surgeon in private hospital. He previously was in government job and took voluntary retirement in 2005. Since 2005, he is in private practice. He has a family history of hypertension. His father (90) has problem of hypertension. However, the respondent is having no chronic disease.

He is following a healthy lifestyle such as regular eating schedule, healthy and balanced diet, regular physical activity, non-consumption of tobacco and alcohol. He is following this lifestyle for last more than 25 years along with a regular practice of yoga every morning. After dinner he goes for small walk. The respondent is very much regular in his intake of healthy and balanced diet. He keeps his meals very light. He always eats homemade food cooked in very less oil. He never eats packaged food as they have lot of unnecessary ingredients which are not good for health. Even at social events he looks for most healthy option like grilled fish or salad.

He takes a good night sleep and has been a strong votary of power nap at least once in a day. He is very social and is an active member of IMA (Indian Medical Association). Moreover, he also engages in social philanthropy, for instance, organizing medical camps, langars etc. In his free time, he prefers to do agriculture related activities which also point towards an active lifestyle. He says "I have never taken a sick leave in my life from work." He says he realizes the importance of good exercise and moderate work out for long and healthy life.

From the above case study, we come to know that healthy lifestyle curbs the development of a disease even it is considered as mainly genetic in origin. Here also a healthy lifestyle is the reason for non development of a chronic health condition.

**Case: 013**

*No chronic illness with family history of Heart Problem and Peptic Ulcer*

*Family History of disease: Heart Problem, Peptic Ulcer*

Dr. Smriti is 65 years old female living in joint family and working in private hospital as a gynecologist. She is doing practice for the last 39 years. She is satisfied with her professional and personal life. She is an active participant in health promotion programs. She is healthy despite having a family history of cardiac problem and peptic ulcer.

She has a very healthy lifestyle right from the beginning. She says "I know the diseases I can get if I don't maintain healthy lifestyle." She has switched to whole grain foods like brown rice, oats, quinoa etc. She has cut down non-vegetarian food. She takes honey or jaggery as a substitute to white sugar. She takes low sodium diet. She eats more fruits, vegetables, low dairy products and other healthy foods at home. She does all kind of physical activities like brisk walk, swimming and other aerobic exercises. She goes for swimming 4 days a week. She says "It was easy to make these small changes which helped her to lead a healthy and happy life"

Though she has to work seven days a week and for more than eight hours a day, she does not consider her work stressful. She enjoys her work. She says "I know stress is breeding ground for all the kind of diseases and it lowers the immunity of a person to fight with diseases. Therefore it becomes all the more important to do exercise regularly and monitor what you eat."

As we know that 'lifestyle related diseases' are also known as 'diseases of longevity', so as the age increases the incidence of development of these diseases also rises especially when there is family history of disease. But in this case even after attaining an age of 65 years the respondent is not having any chronic illness. This reaffirms that genes are not the sole reason for the development of disease, lifestyle is also important for the causation of disease.

## Difficulties Faced by the 'Doctor-Patient' Due to Casual Approach by the Physician

The doctors are supposed to be more careful and aware about their health as compared to an ordinary person. But in reality, it was observed in some cases that not only doctors as patients ignored their health related issues but even the physician treating the 'doctor-patient' took the illness for granted.

Occasionally the health problems of a 'doctor-patient' are not diagnosed seriously by the physician and many queries are left unattended or ignored leading to serious health consequences.

We came across such case where the medical knowledge of 'doctor-patient' was taken for granted and some required tests were not done that lead to development of complications later on.

**Case: 014**

*Callousness by the 'doctor-patient' himself and his physician resulted in a complicated and Chronic Eye Problem.*

*Family history of disease: Negative*

Dr. Dalbir is 47 year old living in nuclear family and working in government hospital. He did his M.B.B.S. in 1996 and joined government hospital in 1998 and completed his post-graduation in 2005. In 2008 he started experiencing blurred vision and redness in his eyes. This was accompanied with poor vision and he was prescribed reading glasses. But still he found himself rubbing his eyes continuously. Initially, he ignored the problem and self treated himself by using eye drops intermittently, but the problem kept on aggravating. In 2010, on the advice of his friend, he consulted the Head of the Eye Department where his problem couldn't be diagnosed properly and was prescribed some other eye drops which relieved him temporarily. However, it resulted in further inflammation and deterioration of vision.

After five years of continuous distress in the year 2013, on being insisted by his family members, he consulted a visiting eye specialist at a private hospital in Ambala. After a thorough check-up, he was diagnosed with severe eye inflammation, cataract and lens deterioration in both eyes and was referred to PGI, Chandigarh for further consultation in October, 2013.

In PGI he was detected with high blood pressure and high cholesterol level along with chronic eye problem. As the case was a complicated one, a team of doctors from AIIMS (Delhi) was called to assist the PGI doctors in his eye surgery.

Thus, initially due to the ignorance and negligence of the 'doctor-patient' and careless attitude of the Ophthalmologist a minor eye inflammation problem became a complicated case that might have led to the permanent loss of vision. The study also reveals that doctors regularly advises the patient to undergo the routine medical check-ups after a certain age but they do not apply this to their own lives as witnessed from this case where the doctor-patient's own problems of hypertension and high cholesterol levels were detected accidentally during the thorough check up of his deteriorating eye problem.

The doctor after undergoing such a bad experience advices, "Never take your health related problem lightly and always take a second, third and even fourth opinion from doctors if situation demands so."

**Lack of Social and Emotional Support System Lead to Development of Disease**

Social and emotional support for individual is an indispensible function of social institutions like family, peers, colleagues. They play an important role in maintaining a congenial environment where an individual reaches his highest physical and mental potential. The absence of this support system often leads to anxiety and stress related disorders which drive individuals towards sedentary lifestyle and risk factors like alcoholism in turn developing lifestyle related disease.

**Case: 015**

*Lack of social and emotional support lead to sedentary lifestyle and alcoholism resulting in Cardiac issues. Death of the wife leads to negligence regarding medical and health care.*

*Family History of disease: Hypertension (Father)*

Dr. Damanpreet is 69 years old male living in joint family and is presently working in private hospital after he got retired from government job in 2007. He is having diabetes and high blood pressure and he attributes this to his sedentary lifestyle which he developed after his wife's death in year 2007 which came as an emotional setback. He was also not able to cope up with the death of his wife. He gradually developed anxiety issues and stress related problems. There was no support system available to him even from his children and colleagues. His lifestyle changed a great deal as home cooked food was replaced by outside food and regular walks with his wife replaced by sitting in home in isolation. He also has a family history of hypertension.

His lifestyle was already inactive and death of his wife made it worse. He started remaining in seclusion and confined himself to his practice and his leisure activities like reading    books, watching television and listening to music. He also started to take alcohol frequently.

He is obese and needs to follow a regular fitness routine along with regular health check-ups which may help him in regaining his physical fitness and increase his life span.

Thus the case study brings out the consequences of lack of emotional support leading to development of health issues. Death of the loved ones, as highlighted in this case, pushed an individual towards a sedentary lifestyle. This consequence could have been averted if the social system of emotional support was available to the patient. The respondent's wife was the only emotional support system for him and after her death this system collapsed resulting in unhealthy lifestyle and development of ailments.

In this case study, genetic history of disease was a non-modifiable risk factor while loss of emotional and social support acted as a trigger for development of the cardiac problem. This proves that social institutions play a key role in stabilizing the individuals and assure their well being.

**Case: 016**

*Emotional traumas and lack of emotional support lead to development of Hypertension, Mild Osteoarthritis and Depression*

*Family History of disease: Father (Hypertension), Mother (Cancer)*

Dr. Kamalpreet is 60 years old female living in nuclear family and working as gynecologist. She has multiple health related issues. She is suffering from hypertension for the past 25 years, mild osteoarthritis for 6 years and severe depression for the past 2 years. In case of hypertension, headache and in case of osteoarthritis knee pain appeared as symptoms. In spite of having so many symptoms she did not make regular visits to her doctor.

She suffered from many emotional traumas in her early life. After the death of her father, she was the eldest of her siblings and suddenly all the responsibilities of her family came to her shoulders. She had issues with her marriage and did not get required support from her husband and his family. She was not involved in important family decisions and was treated secondary in familial matters. She couldn't even control her own salary. All this weighed on her mind. This unsupportive environment caused her to take a lot of stress and anxiety. Due to her family tensions and busy work schedule she was unable to follow healthy diet pattern or indulge in some physical activity because of which she is slightly obese. All these issues together made her cynical and self critical.

She says "It is not easy for me to follow a healthy lifestyle." As far as coping is concerned she finds it difficult to adjust or perform in such stressful environment. Lack of emotional support has caused multiple health related problems which further interfere in her social, recreational, household and professional responsibilities. She feels discouraged, fearful and worried most of the time. Frustration, physical and mental fatigue is frequent and she thinks of taking break from work. It is difficult for her to cope up with her ailing condition and this undermines her confidence on herself and her abilities as a doctor and a home maker.

Thus, this case study points towards many factors like emotional traumas due to death of her father, non-supportive attitude of husband, lack of independence in using her own hard earned money on herself, lack of emotional support by her in-laws etc. At the same time, role of family history of hypertension cannot be denied. Also, the psychological effect and less coping ability is quite visible in this case that reveals that in case of any crisis a social and psychological support system is always desirable, that is missing in this case.

**Too Much Difficulty in Coping Up with the Lifestyle related Disease**

After occurrence of disease, a phase comes when the patient has to manage his or her chronic health conditions by making adjustments in his or her day to day life. Here, we found that there were some cases where respondents found it difficult to make adjustments socially and psychologically.

In the below mentioned case the doctors could not cope up well despite knowing about the disease and she did not take proper medication or exercise. Further, the stress of one disease led to onset of another disease.

**Case: 017**

*Development of Auto Immune Disease (AID) leads to depression and stress which eventually lead to Hypertension.*

*Family History of disease: Hypertension (Father)*

Dr. Gurinder is 49 years old married woman from a joint family system. She is in government job for past 20 years. For the last 14 years, she is suffering from auto-immune disease. Due to which she is allergic to a number of allergens present in the environment. This problem led to the onset of depression and stress which further compounded into hypertension twelve years ago.

She has a family history of hypertension but no family history of auto-immune disease. She refrains from any physical activity due to her problem of frequent allergic reactions making her obese. Adding to this, she is very fond of processed foods. She is now on anti-hypertensive medicine continuously for the last twelve years and also taking anti-allergic medicine on and off.

Social and psychological effects of lifestyle related disease are quite visible in this case. The social, recreational, household and outdoor activities are moderately affected and eating habits are very much affected by the disease. The absence of proper coping mechanisms is evident in the form of discouragement, fearfulness, worry and frustration. Physical and mental fatigue is also experienced by the respondent. The respondent herself is not very confident in coping with fatigue, physical discomfort and emotional distress.

This case study is peculiar because here the respondent took a long period of time to accept and cope up with the illness. Also, stress as a result of an illness gave birth to the other chronic condition. This shows that the respondent was not able to cope up with the situation of crisis due to lifestyle related disease and that resulted in to development of an additional chronic condition. Thus stress due to initial chronic illness catalyzed the onset of other lifestyle related disease.

**FOCUSED GROUP DISCUSSION**

A Focused Group Discussion (FGD) is a research tool that involves a focused debate by participants on a research topic which is often mediated by the researcher. Here, researcher encourages the participants to share their views and experiences on a defined topic.

For making a deeper analysis of lifestyle related diseases among doctors, a Focused Group Discussion was arranged at Service Club in Amritsar. The discussion involved 12 doctors belonging to different areas of specialization from both clinical and non-clinical branches of medical field. The doctors were specialist in Pharmacology, Pathology, Medicine, Gynecology, Eye, ENT etc. The doctors were practicing in both private and government sector.

A brief introduction about the topic of discussion was given to all the participants. After introducing the topic, researcher asked the respondents to express their views on the different aspects of lifestyle related diseases such as;

A. Causes and risk factors associated with lifestyle related diseases

B. Impact of lifestyle related diseases on doctors

C. Experiences of 'doctor-patients' and coping mechanisms adopted to   manage the lifestyle related diseases.

In the Focused Group Discussion, name of the doctors have been intentionally concealed as part of the research ethics.

Conversation started with Dr. A emphasizing that lifestyle related diseases are not uncommon among doctors. He explained "As a general practitioner, I come across a lot of 'doctor-patients' having various lifestyle related health issues, particularly hypertension and diabetes among doctors."

One of the participants Dr. B added that once considered as the diseases of longevity, these diseases are now affecting the comparatively younger age group. "Faulty lifestyle is the major risk factor for the causation of lifestyle related diseases." He remarked.

Most of the participants also shared their concern about the detection of lifestyle related diseases among young people.

Dr. K, who is head of the Pharmacology Department, mentioned that one of his students in his twenties is suffering from hypertension. He explained that irregular diet pattern is common among medical students and medical practitioners.

To this Dr. B added that he works in a private hospital, where the work schedule is very hectic. He takes care of both OPD and IPD sections. He said "In case of emergency duty, I work for both day and night. Due to this busy work schedule, timely intake of food becomes difficult".

Most of the doctors concurred with Dr. K and Dr. B that the doctors are irregular in their diet pattern because of their hectic work schedule.

To this, Dr C added that "not only the irregular meal schedule but also the bad eating habits are a major issue in lifestyles. Invasion of processed fast food culture has added on to this bad habit of doctors".

Majority of the respondents were of the view that like an ordinary person, doctors have tendency to eat processed food and aerated drinks. Dr. K added that even during the medical association meetings the food served is not very healthy. Some of the doctors also said that they generally go outside for dinner on every weekend taking junk or fast food.

Further, Dr. A  said that lack of physical activity among doctors plays a much bigger role as compared to faulty eating habits. "As a doctor I have been dealing with many 'doctor-patients'. The doctor's sedentary lifestyle and lack of any sport activities is the major reason for diseases like diabetes, obesity, high cholesterol etc."

Dr. D, a young M.D, interrupted abruptly that 'work is worship', so the doctor's focus is mostly on treating the patients and the self-care sometimes becomes secondary for doctors.

Most of the doctors participating in Focused Group Discussion said that they are too busy in their professional life to spare time for physical activity. To this, some of the participants added that even if they do have some extra time in their busy schedule, they prefer to watch television or read some books.

Upon this Dr. K commented "No one is too busy to take care of their health. I think doctors are more callous in their approach rather than being busy in their professional life".

Few of the doctors were of the view that being medical professionals they are well aware about the benefit of physical activity but sometimes health related issues and lack of proper weather conditions may become a barrier to physical activity. "The environmental pollution is important factor for discouraging regular walk and exercise among the doctors." said Doctor A.

Dr. E however, said that his Asthmatic condition is a reason for physical inactivity. He said, "My breathing problem restrains me from doing any kind of indoor or outdoor physical activity. There is lot of environmental pollution and I am allergic to dust" Other participant Dr. J suffering from Arthritis supported this argument and expressed her inability to do exercise due to her joint pains.

Dr. F who is a surgeon in a government hospital remarked, "Only during OPD times there is more sitting, otherwise doctors have to move around the hospital for routine check-ups and follow-ups of the patients. I think it is more of stressful nature of job rather than physical inactivity as major cause for lifestyle diseases."

Another doctor Dr. I who is a diabetic patient emphasized that there is high stress associated with the job of the doctor. This sensitive nature of the job along with long work hours and poor physical activity leads to lifestyle diseases. To this, Dr. B added that stress becomes double while working in a private hospital due to lack of job security or regular income. Also, doctors with their own private practice sometimes feel insecure about their income on regular basis. Many of the doctors were of the view that working in government hospital is comparatively easy due to security of job and fixed working hours.

Dr. G added to the conversation another risk factor i.e. consumption of alcohol and tobacco. He is a senior doctor heading a de-addiction center in a government medical college. He stressed "many of the chronic lifestyle diseases are the consequence of excess use of alcohol and tobacco consumption".

Dr G said "I have a vast experience of counseling addicts. Many doctors with lifestyle diseases consult me on their addiction problems. The visiting 'doctor-patients' are addicted to excessive consumption of alcohol in their day to day life".

Another participant, Dr. L, a cardiac patient said that the main reason for my heart attack at a very young age was my habit of cigarette smoking. He further added that he used to smoke 15-20 cigarettes per day.

Many of the participants of the view that use of the tobacco products are harmful but consumption of alcohol in controlled quantity has medicinal value.

Upon deliberation on what should be included in the healthy diet, most of the doctors talked about importance of consumption of fruits and vegetables/legumes on daily basis.

Dr. C informed "there is WHO recommendation of five servings of fruits and vegetables or legumes for a healthy diet". Ironically very few were aware about this recommendation.

Few of the participants mentioned that they are quite aware about the WHO recommendations of healthy and balanced diet. Some other doctors added that they try to consume ample quantity of fruits and vegetables in their diet, but it becomes difficult for them to follow this in routine.

One of the participants, Dr. H, showed resentment by saying that sometimes a person may suffer from a disease even after following a healthy lifestyle. She said that she used to follow a healthy lifestyle but still she suffered from cancer.

The conversation rolled towards the impacts of lifestyle related diseases amongst Doctors. In the Focused group discussion; there were 5 doctors with different lifestyle related diseases. They highlighted the socio-psychological and economic impact due to lifestyle related disease they suffered. All the doctors said as they belong to upper income group therefore they did not face any economic issues as compared to common people.

The impacts were more social and psychological. For instance, Dr. H was a gynecologist and was diagnosed with cervical cancer. She recalls "As soon as the news broke out of the test, I was devastated and started crying in front of the doctor". She was really intense telling her tale. She said "it was very difficult to digest the fact that despite being a professional in curing people, I was helpless in my own case. During the initial days, my social activities were reduced a lot due to chemotherapy. Also, I remained anxious and worried thinking about my small children and what will happen to them when I will be gone. But I was lucky to have good social environment. My friends and family helped me in providing the required emotional support to overcome the stress of disease and fight it back".

Dr. I, who was diagnosed with diabetes, took it pretty well. He said "My medical knowledge made the news of disease more palatable. For just a brief period of time I was fretful but I adjusted with it and started my medication to control my diabetes".

While talking about their experiences as patients, doctors discussed about the coping mechanisms with their respective lifestyle related diseases.

Dr. I stated "The impact of news of my disease was minimal. Both of my parents are diabetic and I was also expecting it in my lifetime. Also, as a medical professional, I was confident that I can manage this problem with right medication and change in lifestyle. I was very fond of sweets and chocolate but now I totally stopped the use of these sweets. I have also joined swimming club and am doing cycling regularly.'

However, in response to the Dr. I statement about the family history of diabetes in his case, Dr. L said that family history is not the only factor responsible for the development of lifestyle related diseases. To justify his statement, Dr. L said," I am heart patient without any family history of heart problem." Majority of the participants suggested that a healthy lifestyle like balanced diet, physical activity etc. are as important as medicine to treat the lifestyle related diseases.

In response to the statement of Dr. I where he mentioned that he felt minimal psychological effect on the diagnosis of diabetes, Dr. L revealed "when I was detected with cardiac problem, I was taken aback as I was the first one in my family to suffer from any kind of heart problem at such a young age. Though I was aware that it is possible to completely manage heart problem with right changes in the lifestyle by taking low fat and low sodium diet and increase the intake of green vegetables and pulses still I felt sometimes insecure about my future. There were bouts of stress, anxiety and restlessness".

Dr. J, suffering from Arthritis said, "Pain in joint restricts the normal social and outdoor activities. Due to the excessive stiffness and pain in joints, especially during winters it becomes very difficult to carry on the normal routine activities". Dr. I added that he also felt sometimes low inclination to go outside due to high level of blood sugar.

While discussing the role of social support system during illness period, most of the participants were of the views that a support system is needed always in the time of crisis. Dr. L, suffering from cardiac problem, told that "the emotional support from friends and family was very crucial in those times and it helped me to lead a normal life again".

Further, Dr. H, a cancer survivor added that "emotional support in times of crisis can help a lot in comforting the patient and the patient feels less alone". Dr. H further says "I am a cancer survivor and was detected with first stage cervical cancer. I felt very anxious and vulnerable but with regular emotional support from family and friends and timely treatment from an experienced specialist I was able to not only defeat cancer but also was inspired to live a healthy lifestyle. I think that a good doctor is next only to god and can save lives".

Being an asthmatic, Dr. E enunciated "Coping up for me was very difficult as asthma requires constant monitoring of one's lifestyle. Initial years were very difficult to adjust. The support of family played a key role in psychological adjustment of my diseased state. Moreover I incorporated various mechanisms in my day to day life. There was a significant change in the dietary pattern after the onset of my disease. For physical activity I started yoga practice and meditation".

During the discussion, there was a general viewpoint that doctors knew very well about the long term effect of lifestyle related diseases and medication on the human body. For example, diseases like diabetes and hypertension have harmful effect on different organs of the body like eyes, kidneys and heart etc. Therefore, doctors become apprehensive about their future health when they suffer from some chronic disease.

While discussing the importance of consulting a specialist for a disease, majority of the participants were in the favor of consulting some specialist rather than self medication. Dr. L said that it is always better to consult a specialist as only a specialist can differentiate between a minor problem and emergency situation. He further added, "When I felt pain in chest, I took it as a muscular pain or pain due to gastritis but after consulting cardiologist I came to know about my heart attack".

Further, Dr. I stated "when I was detected with diabetes, I did not visit any other doctor for my treatment. I took standard medicines to cure his type II diabetes because I already had the family history of diabetes and very well know the line of treatment for diabetes. He further said "So I never felt any need to visit specialist as I had full knowledge about the course of treatment for diabetes and I kept checking his blood sugar level regularly".

But not many doctors approved Dr. I decision of self medication. Dr. J said "Initially, when I had pain in my knee joint, I took it as normal pain due to over work and treated myself with pain killers off and on.  But when the pain persisted for a long period of time and aggravated, then I consulted Orthopedician where I was diagnosed with rheumatoid arthritis.   She stresses that "self-medication should be avoided and is even ethically incorrect."

Dr. K also supported the viewpoint of Dr. L about consulting some specialist for illness rather than self-medication. Dr. K visited his friend who is doctor in other hospital in his city. He says "I prefer visiting my doctor friends because I get priority in appointment as I have a very busy schedule during the day". Most of the doctors told that while consulting a specialist they prefer visiting their acquaintances as it is less time consuming.

But not all were of the same opinion. Dr. L said "I never go to my colleagues or family doctor. I always prefer to visit a doctor who is not personally related to me. He said "doctor- patient relation should be strictly professional. Due to privacy issues I visit other doctors as I am not comfortable discussing my health issues with those who know me personally. To avoid the judgments and stigma I always prefer visiting a physician not related to me". Dr. F also agreed to his opinion. He said "I never prefer visiting my colleagues because their knowledge is at par with me and for my treatment I prefer visiting senior specialists who are not related to me personally".

The discussion then moved to the experiences and problems faced by doctors while treating patients who are also doctors.

Almost all the doctors had experience of treating a doctor as patient. Only Dr. D, who is pediatric specialist, did not have any experience in treating 'doctor-patient'.

Few doctors revealed that they had very good experiences with the 'doctor-patients'. Dr. F said "recently I treated a 'doctor-patient' suffering from liver problem. My patient was very regular with the visits and followed all the instructions carefully". Dr. C also shared a same story of his 'doctor-patient'. He said "The 'doctor-patient' was very serious about his treatment and never missed a follow up visit". He also says "I feel that it is easy to treat 'doctor-patients' as they know the seriousness of the disease and are fully aware of the problems even if they don't follow their doctor's advice properly".

While most of the doctors opened up that it is not easy to treat patients who are doctors. Dr. A said "whenever I come across a patient who is doctor, I face a lot of difficulty in treating him. 'Doctor-patients' ask too many questions and are apprehensive of the physician's medical knowledge. They are also doubtful about the prescribed medication".

Dr. L told "sometimes 'doctor-patients' don't reveal full information about their lifestyle. They conceal information about their daily habits which is a big barrier in treatment of any lifestyle disease". Dr. I shared "many times 'doctor-patients' don't abide by the advice and don't follow the instructions. Sometimes the 'doctor-patients' stop taking medicine at their own will".

The doctors were of the view that it is not easy to satisfy a 'doctor-patient' as due to their own medical knowledge sometimes they are not happy with the line of treatment provided by their own doctor.

Documenting this focused group discussion was a very revealing session. We came to know the views of medical professionals as far as occurrence of lifestyle diseases among doctors were concerned. It brought forward key insights which eventually brought new horizons to the research. Through the session we came to know a multi-faceted view of doctors with respect to various socio-economic and psychological aspects of lifestyle related diseases. Further, we got views on the impacts of lifestyle diseases as well as coping mechanisms taken up by doctors who faced lifestyle related diseases. Moreover we also found views of doctors on the behavior of 'doctor-patients' with respect to lifestyle related diseases.

## SUMMARY

All the above case studies and focused group discussion point towards a number of factors that play an essential role in the development and management of lifestyle related diseases.

Most of the Case Studies and Focused Group Discussion revealed that there is not a single reason at a particular time in life that is responsible for lifestyle related disease rather the reasons are hidden in the life history of an individual. Stresses of early life like anxiety during preparation of competitive exams, or unhealthy lifestyle due to the hectic work schedule in the initial years of job or study period or other unhealthy ways of living life lead to manifestation of lifestyle related diseases. Therefore, development of lifestyle related diseases like cardiac problem, respiratory diseases, diabetes, hypertension, osteoarthritis etc. is not the overnight phenomenon; it takes a long time to develop. Risk factors in the form of unhealthy diet, lack of exercise, excessive use of alcohol, consumption of tobacco products and above all stress of personal and professional life are the key reasons for the causation of disease.

Social and emotional support system plays an important and positive role for maintaining a good health as well as in coping up with the diseases. The lack of social and emotional support system has been observed in some case studies i.e. Case 015 and Case 016 where either due to death of spouse or non supportive attitude of spouse or living alone at a far off place without family led to development of lifestyle related diseases. Moreover, during Focused Group Discussion the participants appreciated the support of family and friends during the time of crisis.

Doctor's medical background sometimes is taken for granted in diagnosing and treating a disease that may result in further aggravation of the health issue, For instance in case study, 014.

Coping mechanism was quit challenging in some cases like Case 017 and for Dr. E who is asthmatic patient. Some respondents found it difficult to deal with the chronic illnesses. They were depressed to know about their health condition. Social and psychological effect of lifestyle related diseases was quite prominent in their life. Thus, the above given case studies and Focused Group Discussion provided us the information regarding the experiences and perception of the doctors as far as the lifestyle diseases are concerned.

**CHAPTER VIII**

**SUMMARY AND CONCLUSIONS**

Lifestyle related diseases are also termed as non-communicable diseases or chronic diseases. World Health Organization reported that 60% of all the deaths globally in 2001 were due to these diseases (WHO, 2002) and this mortality rate is expected to grow to almost 75% in 2020 (The World Health Report, 1998). Further, Popkin (2002) mentioned that these chronic diseases are penetrating more rapidly in developing societies than in the developed societies. Owing to the increase in prevalence of lifestyle related diseases, India is facing double burden of both communicable and non-communicable diseases today.

There are number of risk factors responsible for the onset of lifestyle related diseases like unhealthy diet, obesity, lack of physical activity, excessive use of alcohol etc. These factors due to spread of modern culture are now stretching across countries, regions, cultures and communities. So, these diseases once called as 'diseases of affluence' and prevalent mainly in developed nations are now extending to the developing economies.

However, Lifestyle related diseases are preventable. WHO (2005a) in its report mentioned that eighty percent of heart diseases as well as diabetes and forty percent of cancers can be averted by following a healthy lifestyle.

The present research on the 'lifestyle related diseases among doctors in Punjab' focuses on the causes and consequences of these diseases among doctors. The study also tries to elaborate the experiences and coping strategies used by the 'doctor-patients' and the experiences of the physicians of 'doctor-patients'. The rationale for carrying this study among doctors was to assess the prevalence of these illnesses not only among one of the most affluent and educated section of society but also, the section which has the sufficient access to healthcare services. Moreover, this was an area of interest for the researcher to explore the experiences and coping strategies of doctors as patients in role reversal situation. A state of role ambiguity arises when a person in the position of 'custodian of health care services' become the 'consumer' of the same.

In this situation, doctors' medical knowledge and their equal status in relation to the person treating them makes the consultation problematic. Some try to maintain a control of consultations; others look for the status of ordinary patient while some others want that they are special patients with exceptional needs (White, 2002). Further, doctors are considered as the main pillar of health care services. Health of society depends on the physical wellbeing of doctors. As the guardian of health care services, doctors should be in their optimum health.   Vachon (1995) is of the opinion that if the doctors are unsuccessful to look after themselves physically, psychologically, and spiritually, they cannot be expected to give outstanding medical care to others.   In addition, doctors having a healthy lifestyle can more convincingly suggest the healthy lifestyle choices to the patients (Lobelo, Duperly & Frank, 2009). Thus, health of doctors as well as their healthy lifestyle is indispensable for a healthy society.

Most of the studies done previously on the similar topics in Public Health Departments and Community Medicine were mainly focused on incidence and risk factors associated with the lifestyle related diseases. Social aspects of the problem have rarely been touched and very less literature is available in sociology on the research topic under study.

From sociological perspective, biology is not the only dominant factor in the development of disease but the existing social and economic circumstances responsible for onset of disease must be taken into consideration (White, 2002). John Germov (2009) described the transition from 'Bio-medical model' to 'Social model' and traced the origin of these diseases   in to the societal conditions and factors.

Social structure as well as values, beliefs, norms and lifestyle of a society highlight the nature and causes of illness. This is quite common among the people to observe the health related problems from the point of view of their own cultures and to respond to these threats in conventional ways. This identification of importance of the multifarious relationship between social factors and health characteristics of specific social groups led to the development of medical sociology as a significant area within the broad field of sociology.

Sociology is an academic discipline interrelated to the structure and function of the society. It engages the social processes, statuses and roles of social institutions as well as social behaviors of social groups. But medical sociology is associated with the social aspects of health and illness, social functions of health institutions, social behavior of health recruits etc.

Therefore, in the sociological analysis, there are two theoretical branches dealing in the field of medicine and medical professionals. The first is 'Sociology of Medicine' and the other includes 'Sociology in Medicine' (Strauss, 1957). 'Sociology of Medicine' studies the social structure within medical organization and is mainly concerned with the values, norms, role, status associated with this organization, e.g., relationship of doctor and patients, doctor and nurses, role expectation and role performance by medical fraternity etc. Consequently, it analyzes the medical environment from sociological point of view. Researcher came across a number of studies related to this field of medical sociology like studies by T.K. Oooman (1978), T.N. Madaan (1980), Madhu Nagla (1990) etc. which were mainly based on the comparative analysis of different systems of medicines or status and role behaviors of doctors, nurses etc.

On the other hand, 'Sociology in Medicine' is an approach where a medical condition is analyzed and understood from the prism of social setup. Here along with the medical aspect, social aspect is also considered equally important and the emphasis is laid upon the role of social institutions in the origin, continuation and coping up with the disease. 'Sociology in Medicine' is interdisciplinary field where inputs from sociology as well as medical sciences help in managing the medical condition of individual in a holistic manner.

The present research falls within the domain of 'Sociology in Medicine'. Here role of social factors with respect to the lifestyle related diseases among doctors were analyzed from various dimensions to have a comprehensive understanding of the medical condition and find an inclusive solution for it.

The present work is based on the primary data collected from two selected cities of Punjab i.e. Patiala and Amritsar. For the selection of respondents, Indian Medical Association's (IMA) list of doctors was referred and 20% of the doctors in Amritsar and Patiala list were selected. In all, a total sample of 240 doctors belonging to both public and private domain of practice was taken. The purposive sampling was done to ensure representation to doctors belonging to different areas of specialization. The sample thus contained 100 doctors from Patiala city and 140 doctors from Amritsar city.

The main objectives of the study were to identify the prevalence of lifestyle related diseases and their risk factors among doctors as well as to find out the experiences and coping mechanism adopted by doctors to manage these diseases. The other objective was to compare the lifestyle and risk factors among healthy and unhealthy doctors. Another specific objective was to determine the personal, social, economic and psychological impacts of lifestyle related diseases

For this research work, a combination of qualitative and quantitative technique of data collection was used. Quantitative technique is based on the 'interview schedule' that helped in collecting information related to socio-economic, demographic and professional profile of the respondents and prevalence of risk factors etc. from 240 respondents. For qualitative purpose, 17 case studies were done to have a deeper understanding of research work. These case studies described the perception, reaction and coping strategies used by the respondents for dealing with lifestyle related diseases. In addition, a Focus Group Discussion of 12 doctors was also arranged at Service Club in Amritsar for collection of qualitative data.

An interview schedule was prepared by keeping in mind the aforesaid objectives and questions were asked from respondents to get the related information. Researcher selected the   case studies of both healthy and unhealthy doctors. Case studies of unhealthy doctors were primarily based on the peculiar experiences of doctors as patients related to origin and effect of lifestyle related diseases. There were some unhealthy cases suffering from the chronic diseases with or without the family history of diseases, and the healthy cases with the family history of diseases.

In addition, researcher also came across the cases where the lack of social and emotional support was the prime reason for the cause of lifestyle related diseases and there was the other specific case where the coping up with the chronic illness became very much difficult for the sufferer. In addition to all these diverse types of case studies, researcher also located a case study where doctor as patient had to go through the appalling experience because of the insensitive approach of physician towards diagnosis and treatment of his ailment.

During the Focused Group Discussions, objectives of the study were communicated to the participants and a discussion among the participants was carried on. During the discussion the perceptions, experiences, and view points of the participants related to lifestyle related diseases were noted down.

**FINDINGS OF THE STUDY**

The present study was an attempt to determine the incidence and impact of lifestyle related diseases and to find out the experiences as well as the coping strategies executed by doctors to deal with diseased condition. For this purpose, information through interview schedule, Focused Group Discussion, various Case Studies and reports by WHO, FAO, PGIMER, research articles in journals etc. were incorporated.

The findings of the Study are summarized as follows:

**Incidence of Lifestyle related Diseases among Doctors**

More than fifty percent (54.16%) of the doctors in the sample were suffering from lifestyle related diseases. Most commonly found illness was hypertension followed by diabetes. Among the 130 unhealthy respondents, as many as 73 (56.15%) were found to be suffering from hypertension while 34 (26.15%) doctors were diabetic. Other chronic diseases diagnosed among doctors were heart diseases, arthritis, spondylitis, thyroid, asthma, cancer etc.

The doctors assigned multiple reasons for the onset of their lifestyle related diseases. Most commonly accounted reason reported by 97 (74.61%) respondents was stress. Other reasons were physical inactivity, use of alcohol or tobacco, unhealthy diet, age factor etc.

Most (61.53%) of the doctors came to know about their diseased condition only after the symptoms of the disease were visible, though the other 38.46% of the respondents became aware about their illness during routine check-ups. This finding points towards the absence of regular health check-ups among most of the doctors. As far as the duration or history of illness was concerned, in only 5.38% doctors the history of illness was observed for more than 30 years whereas the history of illness up to 10 years was noted in 67.69% doctors.

Findings revealed that 60.41% of doctors had family history of one or the other type of disease whereas 39.58% doctors had no family history of disease. Family history of lifestyle related diseases was observed in a number of case studies, for instance, Case Studies 01,02, 011 etc. However, there were unhealthy cases with no family history of disease e.g. Case Studies 06, 07, 08 etc. In Focused Group Discussion, similar findings were observed where one of the participants was diabetic with a family history and the other one had cardiac problem without a family history of respective disease.

**Socio-Demographic, Economic and Professional Profile of Doctors**

From the Socio-demographic profile of the respondents, majority (82.91%) doctors were found within the age group of 31 to 60 years and 17.09% doctors above the age of 60 years. Maximum and minimum numbers of interviewed doctors fall in the age group 41-50 and above 71 years respectively.

Most (60.42%) of the doctors were male while 39.58% of the doctors were female. Presence of larger numbers of male doctors than female doctors in the sample explained more inclination of men for science subjects. In Case Studies and Focused Group Discussion also, the number of male doctors as compared to female doctors was high. Majority (95.83%) of the doctors in the sample were found to be from both Hindu and Sikh religion. Nearly 83% doctors were married. Present Study also specified that 55% doctors were from nuclear family structure that illustrates the normal urban trend of small size families.

Regarding the Economic profile of the doctors, it was evident that maximum doctors i.e. 40% were earning between 10-20 lacs per annum, other 32.08% were earning more than 20 lacs per annum and there were only 27.91% doctors earning less than 10 lacs. This finding revealed that medical profession is a profitable profession and most of the doctors were in the high income group.

As far as Professional profile was concerned, it was found that there was large number of doctors i.e. 69.58% from clinical branches of specialization as compared to non-clinical branches (30.41%). Also, doctors working in government institutions (72.08%) were found to be higher in number in comparison to those working in private institutions (27.91%). Most (60.83%) of the doctors were working in both

OPD and IPD domains whereas there were only 17.08% doctors associated with teaching in medical colleges.

More than one third of doctors (38.75%) were working all the seven days in a week without any break. Further, there were nearly one third of doctors (32.91%) working more than eight hours a day. As far as the experience of working years in medical profession was concerned, 92.50% of doctors had been in this profession for nearly 40 years and rest were doing medical practice for more than 40 years.

**Comparison of Profiles of Healthy and Unhealthy Doctors**

In this section, socio-demographic, economic and professional profile of healthy and unhealthy doctors was compared. On comparing the age of healthy and unhealthy doctors, it was found that maximum number of healthy doctors (52.56%) were in the age group 41-50 years whereas maximum number of unhealthy doctors (60.29%) were in the age group 51-60 years. A continuous and sharp increase in percentage of unhealthy doctors in comparison to healthy ones was observed after the age of 50 years that revealed that an increase in age has negative effect on the health.

However, many Case Studies i.e. 002, 003, 006 etc. reported the onset of lifestyle related diseases at comparatively younger age. Also, some Cases like 011, 012 and 013 were found to be healthy even at relatively elder age. Further, there was near about double the number of unhealthy male doctors (86) as compared to unhealthy female doctors (44) suffering from lifestyle related diseases that specified more vulnerability of men in contrast to women to chronic diseases.

Majority of unhealthy respondents were from Hindu (57.25%) and Sikh (52.53%) communities whereas other communities like Muslims and Christians had relatively smaller number of unhealthy respondents (28.57% and 33.33% respectively) in comparison to their healthy counterparts. Also, invasion of lifestyle related diseases was observed in doctors (38.89%) belonging to rural areas. This shows that due to the modern lifestyle all the people from both urban and rural areas are at the risk of having these diseases.

Marital status has also found to be an important factor in determining the possibility of onset of lifestyle related diseases. The study revealed that likelihood to appear these diseases was more in divorcees (66.67%), unmarried (68.57%) and widowers or widows (75%) in comparison to married ones (51.01%). In addition to this, in joint family system larger numbers of healthy doctors (55.56%) were found in comparison to those in nuclear families (37.88%). This shows the loneliness along with the lack of social and emotional support as the major causative factors for the beginning of lifestyle related diseases. In Case Studies 015 and 016 also lack of social and emotional support emerged as main reasons for diseases.

In the economic profile, higher income level appeared to have positive relationship for the causation of diseases. As the income level increased, the percentage of unhealthy doctors increased in comparison to healthy ones. For instance, percentage of unhealthy doctors was found to be more than healthy doctors in higher income group i.e. in 10-20 lacs and > 20 lacs income groups whereas percentage of healthy doctors (55.22%) was more than unhealthy doctors (44.78%) in comparatively lower income group (< 10 lacs).

As explained in the Chapter II, there are basically two branches of medical field i.e. clinical and non-clinical branches. Work culture in clinical branches is considered to be stressful as that of non-clinical branches. When a comparison was done between healthy and unhealthy doctors within these two branches, it was found that in non-clinical branches, there was almost an equal number of healthy (49.31%) and unhealthy (50.68%) respondents whereas in clinical branches, unhealthy doctors (55.68%) were more in number in comparison to healthy ones (44.32%).

Also, percentage of unhealthy doctors (64.18%) working in private institutions was higher in comparison to percentage of unhealthy doctors (50.29%) in government institution. Therefore, stressful work culture in clinical branches as well as in private institutions may also be the reason for diseased condition. Similarly, less stressful working conditions and fixed hours in OPD and teaching job resulted in lower percentage of unhealthy doctors as compared to those of working in IPD and in both OPD and IPD.

Number of years of practice, number of working days in a week and number of working hours in a day also seemed to have effect on the health of doctors. In the present study, it was found that as the number of years of practice increased, the number of unhealthy doctors showed upward trend with respect to healthy ones. Also, unhealthy doctors were more in number among those who worked for seven days a week and more than eight hours a day i.e. 62.36% and 58.23% respectively. Similarly, chronic illnesses were found in Case Studies 003 and 009 where the doctors worked for full week without any break and more than eight hours in a day. Studies by Ingrid Philibert (2005) and Steven W. Lockley et al. (2007) also came up with similar findings of harmful effect of long and continuous working hours on the health of doctors.

**Comparison of Lifestyle and Risk Factors among Healthy and Unhealthy Doctors**

The study has tried to explore the role of lifestyle and risk factors for the causation of diseases among doctors. First of all, perception of doctors about their lifestyle was noted. The doctors had the different perceptions about the lifestyle they were living e.g. sedentary or moderately active or very much active lifestyle.  Only 22% doctors said that they had sedentary lifestyle whereas 78% doctors were of the view that they had moderately active or very much active lifestyle.

However, sedentary lifestyle was found to be more common among unhealthy doctors (62.26%) as compared to healthy ones (37.74%). Presence of moderately active lifestyle among 60% of unhealthy doctors suggested that unhealthy doctors were trying to follow a healthy lifestyle to regain health. Among doctors with very much active lifestyle, number of healthy doctors was approximately four times (30) as that of unhealthy ones (7). Similarly, study by Jardim et al. (2015) and Case Studies 002, 007, 008, 015 also mentioned sedentary lifestyle among doctors as one of risk factors for lifestyle related diseases.

There are mainly four risk factors given by WHO for the emergence of lifestyle related diseases such as unhealthy diet, physical inactivity, consumption of tobacco and excess use of alcohol. Along with these four factors, researcher also tried to explore the other factors present in  day to day life of doctors. These factors related to sleeping habit, perception about job, regular health check-ups, leisure activities etc.

may tell a lot about health behaviour of a person. The study revealed important relation between health and lifestyle of doctors.

*Diet*

As per the findings of our study, majority of doctors (75.83%) had regular meal schedule whereas a small number had irregular meal schedule (24.16%). However, doctors with irregular meal were found to be mostly unhealthy (74.13%). Irregular food habits had also been observed in unhealthy Cases 002, 003, 005, 009, 010. Thus, irregular meal schedule was found to be harmful for the health of people.

Further, the doctors irregular in their meal schedule gave multiple reasons for the irregularity. Most (79.31%) of the doctors in interview schedule as well as in Focused Group Discussion assigned the busy schedule as the most common reason for irregular meal schedule. The other reasons were lack of appetite, carelessness etc. In the present study, Cases 003, 005 and 010 also reported one or more than one reason for their irregular meal schedule.

As far as the habit of dining out was concerned, those who never dined outside were found to be healthy and double in number (10) as compared to unhealthy doctors (5). Those who dined outside either frequently or occasionally were found to be unhealthy in higher number as compared to healthy ones. Unhealthy Cases 003 and 004 had the habit of dining outside and also in Focused Group Discussion, majority of the doctors mentioned about their habit of dining outside.

In addition, habit of intake of junk food was observed among almost 82% doctors in the study. A positive relationship between frequency of junk food intake and percentage of unhealthy doctors was observed that shows the negative effect of junk food on the health of doctors. Cases 004 and 008, who were unhealthy, also mentioned the habit of frequent intake of junk food. In addition to these findings, lack of required consumption of milk and milk products was more recurrently observed among the unhealthy doctors.

WHO (2003) prescribes a daily intake of 400 grams or 5 servings of fruits, vegetables or legumes per day. But Department of Women and Child development (GOI, 1998) specified the low intake of fruits and vegetables (120-140 grams) among Indians. A significant finding was viewed among unhealthy doctors regarding intake of ideal quantity of fruits, vegetables or legumes as per WHO guidelines. More inclination in consuming this required quantity was found among unhealthy doctors as compared to healthy ones. Also, in Cases 003, 004 and 008 low intakes of fruits, vegetables or legumes were mentioned. There was shocking revelation in Focused Group Discussion where all the participants did not know the prescribed quantity of fruits, vegetables or legumes by World Health Organization. Some other participants despite knowing the importance of required quantity were not consuming these on daily basis.

### *Physical Activity*

A regular physical activity is required to maintain an optimum body weight. The findings of the present study revealed that 52.92% doctors were either overweight, obese or severely obese and the number of unhealthy doctors (56.64%) with higher body weight is more in comparison to healthy ones (43.36%). However, presence of more than standard body weight was also observed among healthy doctors (43.36%) and it pointed towards the future possibility of emergence of chronic diseases among healthy doctors also. It is relevant to mention here the study by Jardim et al. (2015) and Case Studies 004, 005, 007, 0015 etc. where high incidence of overweight and obesity among doctors were reported.

Moreover, Physical inactivity has been enlisted as one of the risk factors for the emergence of lifestyle related diseases by World Health Organization. Findings of the present study regarding regular physical activity suggested that only 56.67% of doctors were doing regular physical activity whereas remaining doctors (43.33%) were not regular in physical activity. Many Cases i.e. 001, 003, 004 etc. as well as studies by Wada et al. (2011) and Whisker (2012) reported low physical activity among physicians.

Next, multiple reasons were given by the doctors for their lack of physical activity. Busy schedule (65.38%) was felt as one of the most common hurdle against physical activity. Some doctors mentioned too much tiredness (27.88%), lack of interest (23.07%), health related issues (23.07%) etc. as possible reasons for their physical inactivity. Cases 003 and 016 too felt busy schedule as the reason for their physical inactivity whereas in Case 009, health related problem and in Case 010, lack of time was the main cause for lack of physical activity. In Focused Group Discussion, reasons given for physical inactivity were busy schedule, lack of time, health issues, lack of practical conditions like suitable weather etc.

Further, respondents came up with multiple responses as far as the choice for physical activities was concerned. The most favored (62.50%) physical activity among doctors was walking. The other preferred exercises were stretching or strengthening (41.17%), bicycling (13.23%) and swimming (5.14%). Healthy doctors (73.21%) chose stretching or strengthening exercises whereas unhealthy doctors (64.70%) were preferably doing walking as physical activity.

### Consumption of Tobacco Products

Consumption of tobacco products is considered to be harmful for the health of people. Findings suggested the prevalence of use of tobacco products among 24.17% of doctors. Study by Wada et al. (2011) also reported the smoking habit among doctors in Japan. Among those consuming tobacco products, 62.07% were unhealthy and 37.93% were healthy.

Further, in Focused Group Discussion, many of the participants believed that tobacco consumption may be the reason for lifestyle related diseases. Also, Cases 001, 002 and 004 blamed cigarette smoking as the reason for their hypertension and cardiac problem.

### Consumption of Alcohol

The present study found that 41.67% doctors were consuming alcohol whereas 58.33% were non-alcoholic. Negligible difference in number was found among healthy (68) and unhealthy (72) doctors who were not consuming alcohol. However, 58% unhealthy and 42% healthy doctors were found among those consuming alcohol. The presence of more numbers of unhealthy doctors as compared to healthy doctors consuming alcohol shows the damaging effect of alcohol consumption on health.

Similarly Wada et.al (2011) highlighted the habit of alcohol consumption among doctors working in Swiss primary care and Jardim et al. (2015) explored a relation between alcohol consumption and emergence of heart diseases among physicians. Also, Cases 001, 002 and 004 had the habit of alcohol consumption and were reported to be unhealthy. Majority of the doctors in Focused Group Discussion were in the favor of controlled quantity of alcohol as it has medicinal value.

Recommended quantity of Alcohol according to WHO (1999) is two standard units or less than two standard units with minimum two dry days in a week. Out of 100 doctors consuming alcohol, 42 were healthy and 58 were unhealthy. Out of 42 healthy doctors, 24 (57.14%) refrained from alcohol for more than one week whereas among 58 unhealthy doctors, 30 (51.72%) were consuming alcohol almost every day. Those refraining from alcohol more than a week were mostly healthy (85.71%) and among those consuming alcohol almost every day were mostly unhealthy (93.43%). Case 001 was consuming alcohol for four days or more than four days in a week and found to be unhealthy.

As already said, WHO prescribed 2 or < 2 standard units of alcohol. One standard unit contains 10 grams of pure alcohol. As per our findings, 38% of doctors were consuming alcohol with in permissible limit and it was also found that with the increase in quantity of alcohol beyond two units, there is an increase in number of unhealthy doctors with respect to healthy ones. Case 001 had excessive use of alcohol and was unhealthy.

Further, while exploring the duration for taking alcohol, it was found that as the number of years of alcohol consumption increased, there was larger number of unhealthy doctors as compared to healthy ones. For instance, among 25 doctors taking alcohol for 10 years, 22 (88%) were healthy and 3 (12%) were unhealthy and for those consuming alcohol for more 40 years, all (100%) were found to be unhealthy. In Case 004, the doctor consuming alcohol for 20 years was suffering from cardiac problem.

Moreover, there is an interesting finding that intake of alcohol increased among 72.72% healthy doctors whereas its quantity decreased in 90.90% unhealthy doctors. This shows that the unhealthy doctors tried to follow a healthy lifestyle to manage their chronic conditions.

Therefore, all the findings related to alcohol consumptions revealed that alcohol intake more than a permissible limit and for long duration of time had a harmful effect on the health.

*Other Lifestyle related Factors*

In this study, a number of other lifestyle related factors like sleeping habits, leisure activities, routine medical check-ups, perception about sociality etc. had also been explored in order to determine the lifestyle of doctors. The findings related to these aspects are thus discussed.

Sleep is an important reason for the physical and mental health of an individual. Daily requirement of sleep for an adult is 7-8 hours (National Heart, Lung and Blood Institute, 2011). This minimum required sleep reported to be missing among doctors, for instance,  studies by Philibert (2005) & Lockey et al. (2009) highlighted the problem of sleep deprivation among doctors.

As mentioned earlier, Gottlieb et al. (2005) found a positive relationship between lack of sleep and diabetes and Kasasbeh et al. (2006) revealed lack of sleep as the reason for heart diseases and hypertension.

It was found in our study  that most of the doctors (64.17%) had less than 7 hours of sleep whereas 6.67% of doctors had more than 8 hours of sleep. In both the cases, number of unhealthy doctors was more than healthy ones. Also, study by Ayas et al. (2003) revealed the prevalence of higher risk for diabetes and cardiac diseases due to both short and long duration of sleep.

Further, majority of the doctors (76.67%) believed their work as moderately or very much stressful whereas rest 23.33% doctors considered their work not at all stressful. A number of studies like Menon & Munalula (2007), Wond (2008), Huggard & Dixon (2011), Govender et al. (2012), Tuthill et al. (2013) and Cases 003 and 013 highlighted the stress at work place among doctors.

Moreover, stressful working conditions may have negative effect on the health. It is evident in our study also. There were more numbers of unhealthy respondents in comparison to healthy ones who considered their work stressful whereas number of healthy doctors was more when work was not felt as stressful.

Next, role of social interaction in the health of respondents has also been explored. Question related to perception of doctors about their way of life. It was found in our study that 66.67% doctors were gregarious whereas 27.08% were solitary in their respective lives. Those living gregarious life were healthier whereas solitary lifestyle was observed more frequent among unhealthy doctors.

Similar findings were established by Robles & Kiecolt- Glasser (2003) and Everson-Rose & Lewis (2005) where low social ties were associated with the emergence of a number of lifestyle related diseases  like heart diseases, high blood pressure, immune systems etc. Cases 003 and 005 living solitary life had health issues whereas Case 012, gregarious in nature, had no chronic illness even at the age 62 years.

Type of leisure activity performed predicts a lot about the lifestyle of a person. In our study, it was disclosed that majority of the doctors were interested in sedentary leisure time activities like watching television (50.83%) and reading books (44.16%) in their free time. Moreover, number of unhealthy doctors was more in contrast to healthy ones involved in sedentary leisure activities. Unhealthy Cases 003 and 015 also mentioned reading books and watching television as their leisure time activities.

The regular health check-ups illustrate the awareness of the persons about their health. Our findings explained that both unhealthy (27.55%) and healthy doctors (72.45%) were not regular in their routine health check-ups. However, unhealthy doctors were found to be more frequent in health check-ups in comparison to healthy doctors. Similarly, irregularity in health checkups was reported by Cases 001, 003, 006 and 008.

**Impact of Lifestyle related Disease on Doctors**

Livneh and Antonak (1997) highlighted the physical, psychological and social effects of chronic diseases on a person's life. These diseases may affect the quality of life of an individual by influencing the choice of diet, physical activity and existing surroundings of a patient (Newman et al., 2004). The present study explored the impact of lifestyle related diseases on personal, social, economic and psychological conditions of 130 unhealthy doctors.

*Impact on Personal Life*

The findings of the study suggested that a diseased person's life got affected on different fronts.  These diseases shaped the routine and outdoor activities as well as the eating habits of the diseased. In case of interference with the routine activities, these diseases affected the activities of 51.53% doctors whereas other 48.46% reported no interference with their routine activities. Also, Case 010 suffering from rheumatoid arthritis and study by Volpato et al. (2002) in diabetic patients highlighted the effect of diseases on the routine activities.

After discussing the effect of chronic diseases on outdoor activities, it was found that 51.53% of doctors felt an interference whereas the remaining 48.47% felt no interference with their outdoor activities. It is relevant to mention the Case 004 and Case 005. Case 004 reported moderate impact on outdoor activities whereas Case 005 increased the recreational activities to deal with the diseased condition. In similar way, Dr. E (Asthmatic) and Dr. J (patient of Arthritis) had to restrain their outdoor activities due to their chronic diseases and Dr. I also discussed the low inclination to go outside in case of raised blood sugar level.

As far as the impact on eating habits due to ailing condition was concerned, 88.46% doctors felt an effect on their eating habits which illustrated the willingness to change the eating habits by diseased person. Changes in eating habits were visible in Case Studies 001, 006 and 009. Case 001 mentioned few changes in eating habits, Case 006 decreased the use of junk food and Case 009 reduced the intake of sodium and fat and preferred home cooked food after the onset of cardiac problem. Similarly, in Focused Group Discussion, Dr. L discussed the effect of cardiac problem on his eating habits that resulted in following a healthy diet schedule and Dr. I, a diabetic patient, had to follow a strict diet plan due to the diabetes.

### Impact on Social Life

Impact on social life includes not only an effect on social ties with family, friends or neighbors but also a feeling of stigma in social system. The findings of the study revealed that though 47.69% of doctors felt no effect on their social life but an impact was felt by 52.30% doctors on their social life. The study by Royer (1998) also specified that chronic illness resulted in less social interaction. In Case Studies 001, 005, 009, 010, 016 very much effect on social interaction was reported whereas in Case Studies 002, 003, 004, 006, 007, 008, 017 effect on social life was moderate. Similarly, effect on social life was observed in Dr. H, suffering from cervical cancer. She mentioned that initially due to chemotherapy her social activities were curbed for a short period.

According to Weiss et al. (2006), social impact of illness includes stigma as an important component. This feeling of stigma was absent in 92.30% doctors that suggested the Stigma is generally not felt due to non-communicable physical illnesses. No one in the Case Studies as well as in Focused Group Discussion mentioned feeling of stigma due to the diseased condition.

### *Economic Impact*

Economic cost of disease was estimated by analyzing the both direct and indirect cost of disease. Direct cost is calculated by expenditure incurred on medicines, tests etc. and indirect one is estimated in terms of effect on efficiency of work and absence from work.

The present study found that 83.07% doctors felt no direct or very low cost of illness because of their good economic condition, treatment on discounted rate or medical reimbursement. No one in Focused Group Discussion and Case Studies reported to be much concerned for direct cost of disease. This confirms that doctors are in good economic condition to meet expenses incurred on illness. In the present study, majority (86.92%) of the doctors reported to spend the money out of their pocket for treatment.

In case of indirect cost of illness, the study found that 36.15% doctors had never took break from work whereas 54.61% took break but sometimes and 9.23% doctors said that they had break from work mostly. This informs that 54.61% doctors had not taken frequent break from work and only 9.23% doctors took recurrent break from work. It is imperative to mention here that the doctors who took break from work sometimes or mostly had to suffer an economic loss due to this break. But, Cases 006 and 016 were interested to take break from work due to their illnesses.

Further, effect on the efficiency of work due to illness may result in economic loss. On exploring the effect of illness, it was found that 50% of the doctors felt no effect on the efficiency of work, 46.92% of the doctors reported the effect sometimes. There were only 3.07% doctors who said that their efficiency was affected frequently or mostly. This shows that efficiency at work got affected due to chronic illness. In Case 004 also, an effect on efficiency of work was noticed.

### *Psychological Impact*

As already said lifestyle related diseases are of long term duration and are never completely curable. These chronic conditions require medication for rest of life along with the change in lifestyle. The modifications in lifestyle include adjustments with the eating habits, social obligations, routine activities etc. Moreover, continual medical condition and constant intake of medicines for a long period may have complications in later life. This type of confined life as well as apprehensiveness of future health put a lot of pressure on the psychological condition of patient. Turner and Kelly (2000) also mentioned that chronic illnesses demand lifestyle related changes and treatment for a long period that result in to emotional traumas among the people suffering from diseases.

In our study it was found that psychological condition of the doctors got affected due to the lifestyle related diseases. Various kind of feelings like feeling of discouragement, fearfulness, worry etc. were mentioned by the 'doctor-patients'.

As far as the feeling of frustration was concerned, 50.76% of doctors had no feeling of frustration while 31.53% had this feeling sometimes and 17.71% had it mostly.

Feeling of discouragement is related to loss of inner confidence to deal with the disease. Among the 130 unhealthy doctors, it was found that 36.15% doctors never had feeling of discouragement. There were 54.61% doctors who had sometimes and 9.23% doctors had mostly the feeling of discouragement.

Uncertainty about the future health leads to a feeling of fearfulness among sufferers. Being medical professionals, doctors have the understanding of medical complications of chronic illness that may generate a feeling of fearfulness. This was seen in our findings also. There were 73.84% of doctors who had a feeling of fearfulness whereas 26.15% of doctors did not have this type of feeling.

Worry is commonly felt on the detection of a disease of chronic nature. Our findings of study regarding this feeling among doctors suggested that 31.53% of doctors never had a feeling of worry whereas 56.92% of doctors were worried 'sometimes'. There were only 11.54% doctors who mostly had feeling of worry.

Further, physical and mental fatigue is found to be common in lifestyle related diseases. The study showed that majority (72.30%) of doctors had the feeling of fatigue whereas no feeling of fatigue was visible among 27.69% of doctors.

Findings of the present study revealed the feeling of fearfulness as the most frequent emotion felt by doctors and it is reported by 73.84% doctors and the least commonly found emotion was the feeling of frustration accounted by 49.24% of doctors.

Further, Case Studies 001, 002, 003 felt a number of mixed feelings like fearfulness, discouragement or worry etc. Case 007 found to have slight whereas Cases 008, 009, 010, 017 had considerable psychological impact due to their chronic health conditions.

Similarly, during Focused Group Discussion Dr. H (cancer survivor), Dr. L (cardiac patient) and Dr. E (asthmatic patient) discussed a significant psychological impact whereas Dr. I (diabetic) did not feel much impact on psychological condition due to their health related issues.

**Experiences and Coping Mechanisms**

The present research further looked in to the experiences and coping strategies chose by doctors to recover from ailing condition. The experiences have been analyzed from two angles-first, from the angle of doctor as patient and secondly, from the angle of physician of the 'doctor-patient'.

*Experiences of 'Doctor-patients'*

When a doctor becomes patient, he may have a variety of experiences. These experiences can be different from an ordinary person suffering from disease. The experiences are related to the nature of feeling on detection of disease, satisfaction or dissatisfaction with the behavior of medical consultant etc.

The experience related to the feeling on the detection of disease was reported to be normal by 60% of doctors whereas rest 40% doctors had a feeling of shocked, apprehension etc. Most commonly felt feeling was apprehension (46.15%) for future health and least felt emotion was depression (19.23%). In Focused Group discussion, Dr. H, Dr. L and Dr. J got emotionally disturbed on the detection of their respective chronic diseases whereas Dr. I and Dr. E felt normal.

Also, a sense of disturbance like depression, apprehension and shock prevailed among doctors on the detection of lifestyle related diseases in Cases 002, 004, 006, 009, 010. Similarly study by Mckevitt & Morgan (1997) revealed parallel feelings among physicians.

Further, for the treatment, 73.84% unhealthy doctors consulted some specialist while 26.15% preferred self-medication. In Focused Group Discussion, majority of doctors favored the treatment from specialist doctors, for instance, Dr. L, Dr. J and Dr. K preferred to visit a doctor in their health related problems But Dr. I self-medicated in diabetes.

In contrast to above findings, studies by Laskari et al. (2010), Montgomery et al. (2011) and Schulz et al. (2016) divulged the high incidence of self-treatment among physicians. Self- medication was also chosen by Case 014 for treating the chronic illness.

As far as the familiarity with the specialist was concerned, most (52.08%) of the doctors were interested to go to unfamiliar specialist and a significant number (47.91%) of doctors favored familiar specialist for treatment. In Focused Group Discussion, most of the doctors were interested to consult some familiar specialist in order to save time. Study by Harris (2003) also noted an inclination towards familiar doctors among patients.

Further, for the choice of familiar specialist, 60.86% doctors chose colleague, 32.60% preferred friend and remaining 6.52% consulted relative for treatment.

According to Shabbir et al. (2016) and Asif et al. (2019) there is a close relationship between excellence of healthcare services and contentment of patient. Patient's satisfaction plays an important role in better health outcomes. In the study, it originated that 83.33% of 'doctor-patient' were satisfied and 16.67% were dissatisfied with physician's behavior. On exploring further, a variety of reasons were given for both satisfaction and dissatisfaction. Most common reason for satisfaction (27.50%) was the sincerity with which their illness was dealt in first visit and laxity in diagnosis of disease was the most frequent reason for dissatisfaction (37.50%) with the treatment. Negligence in diagnosis and treatment was also complained by Case 014 due to which his illness got aggravated.

### *Experiences of 'Physician' of 'Doctor-patient'*

After looking in to the experiences of doctor as patient, out next interest was to find out the experiences of physician while treating a 'doctor-patient'. The present study revealed that 199 (82.91%) doctors out of total sample of 240 doctors had the experience of treating a 'doctor-patient' in their lifetime. In Focused Group

Discussion, almost all the doctors treated the 'doctor-patients' except one doctor who was child specialist.

However, 75.87% physicians said that treating a 'doctor-patient' was difficult, 12.06% found 'doctor-patient' easy to treat and for 12.06%, treatment experience is just like routine patients. During Focused Group Discussion, most of the physicians were of the view that doctors as patients are difficult to treat but few physicians mentioned pleasurable experience of treating 'doctor-patients'.

Further, reasons for difficulty in treating 'doctor-patients' were explored. The findings disclosed many reasons that make 'doctor-patients' difficult to treat. It was observed that compliance is poor among 'doctor-patients'. Only 40.20% physicians told that doctor as patients always show compliance, 53.76% physicians found the compliance with their advice occasionally and no compliance was reported by 6.03% physicians during treatment of the 'doctor-patients' .

Doctors as patients were also found to be irregular in their treatment. More than half of the physicians (54.27%) believed that doctor as patients occasionally came for follow-ups whereas 30.15% physicians confirmed the follow-up visits frequently and 15.57% were of the view that doctor as patients never come for regular follow-ups during treatment. Therefore, 69.84% 'doctor-patients' were not regular in their visits to doctors. In Focused Group Discussion, many doctors had highlighted diverse reasons for difficulty in treating 'doctor-patients', for instance, very much anxiousness or inquisitiveness regarding chronic health condition, concealing the details of disease or non-compliance with doctor's advice etc.

### *Coping Mechanism among Doctors*

According to Compas et al. (2001) coping is, "conscious and volitional efforts to regulate emotion, cognition, behavior, physiology, and the environment in response to stressful events or circumstances." To cope up with the illness, different strategies are executed by doctors like taking the medicine, changing the lifestyle, to pursue leisure activities, doing yoga etc. The present study revealed that 73.97% doctors were regular whereas 26.03% were irregular in taking medicines for high blood pressure. Further, out of 34 diabetic patients, 28 (82.35%) were regularly and 6 (17.64%) were not regularly taking medicines. For other chronic conditions, 69.23% doctors were regular and 30.79% were irregular in taking medicines. Therefore, majority of doctors were regular in taking medicines for various chronic diseases.

Similarly, most of the Cases reported regular intake of medicines in the chronic conditions. Moreover, regarding choice about the form of medicine for treatment, majority (77.69%) trusted Allopathy form of medicine, 13.07% trusted homeopathy and 9.23% preferred Ayurvedic medicine for treatment. All the doctors in the sample are Allopathic doctors, so they preferred to have Allopathic treatment for their illnesses.

Regular health check-ups are essential to identify the disease at an early stage among healthy people whereas among the unhealthy ones, these regular check-ups are required to detect the present status of health. The findings of our study suggested that majority of the doctors (79.23%) were regular in their health check-ups but Case 003 mentioned the lack of regular health check-up even after the detection of hypertension at a very young age.

Further, in case of frequency of health check-ups, it was observed 53.39% 'doctor-patients' had their health check-ups once a year, 33% got their health check-ups done 2-3 times per year and only 13.59% were going for regular health check-ups more than three times per year. Thus, most of 'doctor-patients' (53.39%) had health check-ups at least once in a year.

As origin of lifestyle related diseases is traced to the faulty lifestyle, so the change in lifestyle as well as preventative measures is desired to curb these diseases. In our research findings, it was monitored that 53.84% unhealthy doctors coped up with their diseased condition by changing the lifestyle mostly whereas 45.38% doctors altered their lifestyle sometimes. Only 1 (0.76%) unhealthy doctor denied any change in lifestyle for managing his illness. Though in Focused Group Discussion, majority of the participants were in favor of change in lifestyle to manage the lifestyle related diseases but Case 009 found it difficult to alter the lifestyle even after suffering from heart disease.

Moreover, our study revealed that 52.30% doctors mostly took precautions whereas 46.92% doctors did so sometimes and there was only one doctor (0.76%) taking no safety measure to deal with the disease.

Nowadays, yoga is admired as an important therapy for the physical and mental wellbeing as well as to cope up with the chronic illnesses. Eda (2014) specified the valuable role of yoga in reducing stress among people suffering from chronic conditions like COPD and cancer. So, role of yoga in managing stress in the chronic conditions had also been searched in our study. The results showed that 41.53% doctors included yoga and 58.46% did not prefer yoga to cope up with ailing condition. Practice of yoga was observed in Case 012 for last 20 years and he was not having any chronic health condition despite having a family history of disease. Also, in Focused Group Discussion, one of the doctors suffering from asthma preferred yoga and Meditation to cope up with diseased condition.

Similar to yoga and meditation, leisure activities also help in de-stressing the people. Pressman et al. (2009) emphasized the role of leisure activities in releasing tension. This was visible in our study also. Most of the doctors preferred watching television, reading books etc. to relax. Though, a small number of unhealthy doctors (10) were not involved in any kind of leisure activity.

Umberson (1987) recognized the role of family and friends as a psychological support system and disseminator of the important information associated with health care in case of  physical and mental sufferings. The study found that 55.38% doctors felt that family and social ties helped to a great extent in time of physical crisis and 42.30% doctors said that they helped sometimes in coping up with their diseases. Only 2.30% of respondents did not mention any cooperation from family and friends in diseased condition. However, during Focused Group Discussion, majority of the participants valued the role of family and friends in coping up with the chronic health conditions.

After analyzing the both qualitative and quantitative information related to present study, following observations have been inferred:

**MAIN OBSERVATIONS OF THE STUDY**

- Lifestyle related diseases or chronic diseases like heart diseases, diabetes, cancers are not only biological in origin but social factors play an equally important role for the development of these diseases. Prevailing socio-cultural environment and lifestyle related factors both in personal and professional life have determining effect on the occurrence of these diseases.

- Doctors are generally assumed to be healthier community. It is thought that they can least commonly fall prey to diseases in contrast to common man because of their expertise in the field of medicine and awareness of the causes of diseases In the present study, however, it is found that more than half of the doctors were unhealthy which illustrates that lifestyle related diseases are equally present among doctors also. Most commonly found lifestyle related diseases include hypertension, diabetes and heart disease.

- Both qualitative and quantitative findings of the study suggested that family history of a disease is not the sole reason for the occurrence of lifestyle related diseases. The study suggests that an unhealthy lifestyle as well as non-supportive social and professional environment is equally responsible for these diseases.

- The lifestyle related diseases are often known as 'diseases of longevity' and 'diseases of affluence'. This was reaffirmed in the present study also. While the age progresses beyond 50 years, the number of unhealthy doctors is found to be more as compared to healthy ones. Further, high income may escalate a materialistic, luxurious and sedentary lifestyle where the health of an individual is badly suffered. As the income level increases beyond a certain limit, the number of unhealthy doctors was found to be more.

- Incidence of unhealthy lifestyle and risk factors are evenly distributed among healthy and unhealthy doctors. In the present study, it was inferred that doctors usually do not follow a healthy lifestyle. Though most of them were following regular diet pattern but they were not untouched by the unhealthy food habits. They had more or less habit of eating outside, taking junk food, indulged in the habit of taking tobacco products like cigarette and consumption of alcohol. Unhealthy lifestyle was more visible among unhealthy doctors but this unhealthy way of living was also not unusual among the healthy doctors. This demonstrated that healthy doctors were also at the threshold of development of lifestyle related diseases. Similarly, healthy lifestyle had also been observed among unhealthy doctors that explain the endeavors of unhealthy doctors to follow healthy lifestyle to keep them healthy.

- Sedentary lifestyle as well as physical inactivity was also been among the respondents.   Their leisure activities were also of sedentary nature. Most of the doctors had habit of watching T.V. and reading books as their scheduled leisure activities that pointed towards a sedentary lifestyle. This was indicated by an increase in body weight among doctors.

- Stress had been detected as one of the major cause for the chronic illness. This can be illustrated by the presence of more numbers of unhealthy doctors in clinical branches of medical field, in private institutions as well as in IPD and both IPD and OPD. These aforesaid domains of medical field are deemed to have hectic, tedious and stressful work schedule. Moreover, long and exhaustive years of practice, working for whole week without any break and for more than eight hours a day were also observed to be detrimental outcomes for causation of lifestyle related diseases.

- Social interaction and social ties have emerged as an important social support system for the good health as well as for coping up with the illness among doctors. This was evident when the researcher gathered the data related to the marital status, family structure and the respondents' perception about their sociality. The number of unhealthy doctors with single status e.g. unmarried, widow or widower and divorcee were found to be more in comparison to the married ones. Further, doctors who were gregarious in nature and in joint family set up and were found to be healthy as compared to those in nuclear family set up and living solitary life. Moreover, in coping with the illness, support by family and friends had been found to be productive and useful.

- It was observed that the social gradient of lifestyle related disease is shifting towards younger age group and rural population. These diseases once supposed to be occurring in the old age and predominantly in urban areas, are now affecting comparatively the young population and rural locale too. Besides, male doctors were found to be more vulnerable to lifestyle related diseases as compared to female doctors.

- Casual attitude of doctors had also been observed as far as the routine medical check-ups and treatment of illness was concerned. Most of the doctors came to know about their disease after the appearance of symptoms.

- Just like the common man, doctors too had the feelings of shock, apprehension and depression on the sudden disclosure of disease. But this type of response was observed among less than forty percent of doctors and majority of respondents took the disclosure of disease as normal.

- Socio-economic and psychological impact of lifestyle related diseases was observed among doctors but economic effect especially direct cost of illness was found to be negligible. Indirect economic effect such as break from work and effect on efficiency of work was comparatively more visible as compared to direct cost.

- While going through the literature an inference can be drawn about the habit of self medication among doctors. But in the present study, entirely contradictory observation was found where doctors preferred to consult some specialist in their ailing condition. In Focused Group Discussion too, it was found the doctors were in the favor of consulting some specialist. Further, data suggested less inclination for consulting the familiar doctors whereas in Focused Group Discussion, most of the doctors favored treatment from familiar doctor.

- Doctor as patient and physician of 'doctor-patient' has variety of experiences in their respective statues. On the one hand, the feeling of both satisfaction and dissatisfaction was visible among 'doctors-patients' with the behavior of physicians treating them and on the other side, physicians treating the doctor as patients were not satisfied with them because of poor compliance and irregular follow-ups.

- Importantly, it was interesting to reveal the two contradictory viewpoints in the statuses of doctor as patient and that of physician of 'doctor-patient'. In the status of physician of 'doctor-patient', main criticism by physicians treating the 'doctor-patients' was the irregularity in health check-ups by majority of 'doctor-patients' whereas in doctor as patient's role, majority of doctors confirmed that they had regular health check-ups.

- Majority (more than 70%) of doctors coped up with the help of taking medicines and regular health check-ups whereas most of them (more than 50%) managed their lifestyle related diseases by taking precautions, changing lifestyle and with the help of social ties. Role of yoga and alternative form of medicines as coping strategies to deal with diseased condition were not appreciated much by the doctors.

- An interesting observation of the study was witnessing the doctors from non-clinical branches doing practice as general practitioners in OPDs.

In order to have a deeper and better understanding of the outcomes of the present study, following sociological perspectives have been discussed.

## SOCIOLOGICAL PERSPECTIVES

A diseased condition in society can only be holistically understood when seen from multiple dimensions. When we moved from bio-medical model to social model of disease we came to know that cause of any health related problem is embedded in the social fabric of society. Different social perspectives help in explaining the occurrence, impacts and coping mechanisms associated with diseases. In the present study, multiple facets of lifestyle related diseases among doctors can be visualized through these perspectives. The major perspectives include the Structural-functionalism, the Interactionist or Interpretative and Health Lifestyle theory.

### Structural-Functionalist Approach to Lifestyle related Diseases

According to Structural-functionalist perspective, society can be seen as a system made up of many interrelated parts. Each part plays a particular role to maintain the stability and balance in the society as well to integrate the individual with different social roles. So, society consists of a number of different social institutions like family, hospital etc. which guide the social actors to play roles for the continuation of social life.

Healthy individuals are functional for the society. So, every culture or society tries to give a lot of importance to healthcare of individuals. The individuals are taught in family and other institutions to follow healthy lifestyle which includes good eating habits, physical activity etc.

Parsons (1978) explained that the unhealthy individuals are expected to follow 'sick role' which means that they are to take rest, take proper diet, lead a secluded life and avoid unnecessary exertion and activity. All these activities are considered as major part of sick role. The observance of sick role is functional as it finally leads to recovery from diseases and entry back into the active life.

Parsons further defended his concept of sick role and its applicability in case of chronic illness. He stated that sick role concept is also relevant in chronic conditions. In case of the chronic diseases, such as diabetes and hypertension, complete recovery from illness and normal way of life is not possible. According to Parsons, in case of chronic illness, the further degeneration of the body can be checked by following the doctor's expert advice based on scientific knowledge. The patient has to abide by the doctor's advice for rest of his life. Thus, there is dominance of medical system and subordination of patient's autonomy. This results in to re-structuring the sick role concept but under changed circumstances.

Now in this situation, not only realization of obligations got affected but also diseased person's every day rights are also suspended due to illness and replaced by the rights specified for sick role. An impact on routine and outdoor activities as well as on the eating habits of doctors in their daily life has been observed in the present study and the doctors cope up with these impacts by taking precautions and making changes in their lifestyles.

As illness is deviance and hence dysfunction, a person becomes unable to fulfill the required obligations in specific contexts like in the family and at work place. This is evident in our study also where most of the doctor's normal social activities with the family, friends and neighbors got affected due to lifestyle related diseases. Also, illness resulted in to a negative effect on efficiency of work among doctors.

As far as the functional aspect of social networks or social support system is concerned, doctors residing in joint families were found to be healthy as compared those living in nuclear families. Also, the number of unhealthy doctors was more in single status i.e. as divorcees, widowers etc. as compared to those living with their spouses.

Moreover, non-adherence to prescribed healthy lifestyle and lack of availability of social support systems leads to deviance. This deviance can be seen in the form of risk behaviors like alcoholism and smoking. In our study we realized that doctors lacking social and emotional support systems were engaged more in the consumption of alcohol and tobacco to reduce stress induced by their roles. For instance, in case study

015, it was observed that after the death of wife and lack of support from family and friends, the doctor developed the habit of consuming excess alcohol. This alternative lifestyle produces anomie in the form of doctors with diseases. Our study confirms that the incidence of lifestyle related diseases in doctors with deviant lifestyles increased with their practice years.

Stress is dysfunctional for the individual. This is illustrated in our study also. The doctors working in relaxed working conditions were found to be healthy in contrast to the doctors working in stressed working conditions. For example, doctors working in non-clinical branches and only in OPD and teaching domain as well as working for less than seven days a week and not more than eight hours a day are observed to be healthy in comparison to the doctors who worked in clinical branches, OPD and IPD or both as well as worked for whole week and more than eight hours a day.

Further, lifestyle related diseases among doctors create a role reversal i.e. the doctor in itself is a patient. For such issues structural mechanisms are not adequately functional which we realized in the working of physicians who attended these 'doctor-patients'. Most of physicians in our study highlighted that 'doctor-patients' are difficult to treat. Moreover we witnessed the practice of self-medication which again is deviant (against medical ethics) and produces what Robert K. Merton highlights as 'innovative deviance'. Here doctors adhere to the goal of health but go against the prescribed norms of visiting a doctor for treatment.

Therefore, from functionalist view point, healthy lifestyle is a cherished value in society. It is not only prescribed but also revered. It becomes all the more important for doctors in society, because of their functional uniqueness as 'custodians of health in society'. Hence for a society to survive, it can be summed up that doctors healthy lifestyle acts as a functional prerequisite.

**Interactionist or Interpretative Approach to Lifestyle related Diseases**

The interpretative perspective is based upon the concept of social construction of health as discussed by Conrad and Barker (2010). While explaining that reality is a social construction they said that culture is the important determinant in stigmatizing an illness and label it as disability. Culture controls the way the individual perceives illness. It means that the illness experiences are subjective and not objective reality.

Thus, illness experiences are socially constructed and are reflected in the manner the patients divulge their diseases and make changes in the lifestyle to cope up with the diseases.

Further, interactionist or interpretative perspective approach analyses how individual defines his/her situation and what meaning he/she gives to the symbols during an interaction. So, here patient's "subjectivity" regarding the experiences of illness is explored. These experiences have been expressed through the symbols and reflections, the sufferers developed after recognizing their ailing condition. In addition, state of illness affects the interaction of ailing person with the people close to them. This results in to reorganising the activities related to personal and professional life of an individual. This reorganization, thus, helps in coping up with the ailing condition.

The interpretative perspective has been applied in this study to qualitatively understand the phenomenon by taking in to consideration the experience of being sick from patient's perspective, impacts of the lifestyle related diseases as well as the coping strategies adopted by the person to manage these diseases. Moreover, experiences of physician of 'doctor-patient' are also taken in to consideration to understand difficulties faced by the doctor in treating a person with medical knowledge of chronic health conditions. This perspective was materialized by using the structured interview schedule, taking Case Studies and Focused Group Discussion.

While analyzing the impacts, experiences and coping strategies of individuals suffering from chronic conditions, we came to know that perception and interpretation of these feelings varies from person to person. Most of the doctors took the detection of disease normal whereas for others it was quite distressing and shocking. For them it is something unnatural and deviant, which they want to get rid of. Some case studies illustrated the feeling of disturbance on detection of lifestyle related disease, for instance, Case Studies 002, 004 etc.

Similarly, social activities with family, friends and neighbors had been affected with varied intensity. Perception of psychological impact of lifestyle related diseases was also taken differently by different respondents. Some perceived this impact very much whereas some felt negligible impact. As far as the economic impact was concerned, majority of doctors reported it negligible because they were related to upper strata of the society in economic terms. Thus, social class plays an important role in affecting the perception about the economic impact of lifestyle related diseases.

The 'crisis and negotiation period' for chronic illness is not similar for all the ailing individuals. This period can be understood by looking in to the experiences of being patient and then coping mechanism to restore the normalization. Also, experiences of doctor as patient and physician of 'doctor-patient' gives an insider's view to analyze the two diagonally opposite statuses with prescribed roles.

In the present study, we came to know about the experiences of doctor as patient by knowing about their consultation behaviour and perception about the satisfaction or dissatisfaction with the behavior of doctor treating them on one side. On the other side, experiences of physician of 'doctor-patient' were observed in terms of compliance with the doctor's advice and regular follow-ups by the doctor as patient.

Further, different coping mechanisms were used by doctors to deal with the diseased condition. For instance, some relied on the conventional support systems like family and friends and perceive this as an effective way to reduce stress. While the some others took solace in yoga and routine leisure activities to reduce stress due to diseased condition. The role of medicines, routine health check-ups and alteration in lifestyle was also highlighted in the present study for the management of lifestyle related diseases.

In addition to above perspectives, Post-modern and Psycho-social perspectives also seem to be relevant in the present study.

Post-modern approach came in to existence as a result of changes in the economic structure of the society. This modified economic structure resulted in the revival of liberalism where individual is considered responsible for his health. Here, the focus was upon the individual lifestyle and risk factors. This approach presents an individual with wide range of choices to shape his or her life. This perspective in this study is conducive to know the autonomy of an individual in choosing the lifestyle that may be responsible for the development of a lifestyle related disease. Here, we tried to know about the lifestyle of the individual in the form of eating and sleeping habits, physical work out, consumption of harmful products like tobacco and alcohol, type of leisure time activities etc. The lifestyle can be healthy or unhealthy depending upon the lifestyle choices of an individual.

Psycho-social perspective was also found to be applicable in this study. According to this perspective, stress has been assigned as the main cause of diseases and root of stress is traced in to social and interpersonal relationships. In our study also stress is said to be the main reason for the onset of chronic diseases by majority of doctors. In Case Studies 015 and 016, stress induced by lack of social and emotional support resulted in to onset of lifestyle related diseases.

All the perspectives discussed above, such as functionalist, interpretative, post-modernist and psycho-social perspectives are able to throw light on the importance of healthy lifestyle among doctors as in any other category of individuals.

The most suitable perspective which can explain the lifestyle related diseases among doctors however, is Healthy lifestyle theory developed by Cockerham (2005)

**Health Lifestyle Theory**

There has been a continuous debate in (medical) sociology on importance of both structure and agency for health and lifestyle. And, the debate has been centering on the extent to which one or the other is dominant. Those who are in the favor of structure emphasize that   structural conditions are powerful in shaping the individual disposition and behavior whereas proponents of agency highlight the importance of individualism in choosing the behavior irrespective of influence of structure.

When applied to health lifestyle, the question is whether the decisions people make with respect to diet, exercise, smoking, and the like are a matter of individual choice or are primarily created by structural pressure like social class or gender?

Cockerham (2005) explained the health lifestyle theory based on the concept of life chances and lifestyle choices used by Max Weber (1978) and the concept of habitus by Bourdieu (1984).

Max Weber tried to theorize lifestyles by differentiating it from life chances. According to him, life chances are influenced by the socio-economic position of actors, i.e. their class position which is based on the stratification according to production of goods. Lifestyles, on the other hand, are the characteristics of status groups. They depict the cultural status of the individuals and are based on the basis of mechanism of consumption i.e. styles of life.

Weber tried to analyses the social life through life choices and life chances. Life choices are concerned with choosing from multiple behavioral options while life chances refer to structural probabilities of realizing ones choices. The lifestyles emerge as a result of the dialectical interplay of life choices and life chances.

Bourdieu used the concept habitus. Habitus is a cognitive map or set of perceptions that routinely guides and evaluates a person's choices and options. Individual dispositions toward action are produced by interaction of life chances and life choices.

Thus it is important to understand internalization of class conditions and their transformation into personal dispositions toward action. Individuals who internalize similar life chances share the same general habitus.

According to Bourdieu, habitus is nevertheless an open system of dispositions that is constantly subjected to experiences, and therefore constantly in a mode of modification or reinforcement. The dispositions lead to practices and these practices thus resulted from habitus may be founded on instincts, habits or intentional computation. Bourdieu discussed that these health lifestyle practices may become a part of daily behavioral pattern in such a manner that they are followed automatically e.g. smoking, exercise.

According to Cockerham (2005) lifestyles and structure influences i.e. social class are closely related. General trends responsible for rise in importance of lifestyles in understanding the lifestyle related diseases are;

**a) Transition from infectious diseases to chronic diseases**

In pre-transition period absence of disease was health. So, to avoid the infectious diseases, pathogens and the places inhabited by the infections were avoided but with time due to the development of medical science, improvement in public infrastructure and economic developments, the infectious diseases decreased and possibility of chronic diseases increased. Due to this epidemiological shift from infectious to chronic diseases, the importance of lifestyles came forth.

Previous definition of health where absence of disease considered as health was now replaced by the social, emotional and psychological wellbeing. So, now maintaining a good health is not outside of an individual but it is intrinsic phenomenon by which a person can remain healthy by following a healthy lifestyle. A person has to work consciously to remain healthy.

**b) New modernity in doctor-patient relation**

In this era, a number of new changes occurred in the society. The doctors who used to enjoy a high prestige and status, were no more in this position now. Doctor-patient relationship changed. There was equal distribution of power and decision making between doctor and patient. This was due to the easy access of patients to the information related to  medicine in various web sources available on internet. The increase of uncertainty related to health issues also gave an individual more autonomy to adopt a lifestyle to maintain a good health. But to follow a healthy lifestyle resources are needed. In such a scenario, the social factors become very much significant especially when nature and cause of disease is unidentified.

**c) The transformation of self-identity**

The focus of self identity changed in the present era. Earlier, a person's position in socioeconomic hierarchy was determined by the occupational structure i.e. mechanism of production.  With the rise in market society in 20th century, the patterns of consumption have replaced the mechanism of production as a determinant of the social position of a person. As the lifestyle is reflected in patterns of consumption so it became very important concept in study of health and illness both at the individual level and societal level.

As already mentioned, Cockerham (2000a) defines health lifestyle as "the collective patterns of health related behaviour based on choices from options available to people according to their life chances." Now, life chances are analogous to social structure and life choices are proxy to agency and choices are constrained or enabled by the structure. So, life chances influence the possibility of findings the good things in life by providing the life choices.

The life chances or structural variables are visible in a) social class b) age, gender, race or ethnicity, c) living conditions and d) collectivities. Thus lifestyle choices are determined by these categories. These categories provide the agenda for choices and code of choosing. Socio-economic status, age, gender roles, shared norms and ideologies, neighborhood play an important role in shaping the lifestyle of a person and thus, health lifestyle.

The people belonging to higher income group are in an advantageous position to collect information about new health risks and have resources to adopt new health strategies and practices to maintain a healthy lifestyle. This action (or inaction) in order to maintain a particular health regime leads to its imitation or nullification as well as alteration, by the habitus with the help of a feedback process.

Cockerham believes health lifestyles are of a binary nature, positive and negative depending upon the lifestyle choices. Lifestyle choices may be healthy and unhealthy. The healthy lifestyle includes the health promotion activities like healthy diet, physical activity etc. and unhealthy ones are use of tobacco and alcohol, unhealthy diet etc. These lifestyle choices may be positive or negative and are characteristics of not only individuals but also of whole group sharing the same life chances. The lifestyle reproduces itself over time and these is possibility of make some behaviour changes i.e. selection of some other options according to the life chances but lifestyles remain relatively consistent over time, only open to some degree of change but remarkably durable.

Therefore, healthy lifestyles are individual responsibility but this is constrained by social structure in the form of life chances. Since all the individuals are not equally equipped by the resources i.e. people with better social and economic resources are in a position to adopt healthy lifestyles whereas others are not.

We have seen in our study too that the doctors as a class have better life chances than other category of individuals in the society. This is evidenced by the fact that most of the doctors who follow a healthy lifestyle i.e. doing physical exercise, get routine check-ups, take proper sleep and have availability of extensive support systems like family, friends have lesser prevalence of lifestyle related diseases. We came to know that sedentary and solitary lifestyle, irregular meal schedule, lesser intake of fruits, vegetables or legumes than prescribed quantity, lack of regular physical activity, tobacco use and excessive consumption of alcohol, lack of sleep, stress in job etc. have detrimental for the health of doctors.

## SUGGESTIONS TO PREVENT, MITIGATE AND COPE/ADAPT TO THE INCREASING PREVALENCE OF LIFESTYLE RELATED DISEASES

After analyzing the above findings and observations, following suggestions have been given to avert, alleviate and cope up with the lifestyle related diseases for people in general and for doctors in particular:

### Suggestions for General Public

Public health measures especially at the primary level and awareness among the people are the key factors to address this issue. Here are some suggestions for people in general to prevent and cope up with the lifestyle related diseases. These propositions are as follows:

### *Generation of Awareness*

The first and foremost step should be to create awareness among people about the causative factors and various risk factors responsible for the lifestyle related diseases such as unhealthy diet, excessive use of alcohol, tobacco consumption and physical inactivity etc. The awareness can be carried with the help of social media, by organizing public lectures, by door to door canvassing etc. Even, this kind of awareness campaign can also be carried at school level and at work places to sensitize the people.

### *Free Health Check-ups*

Health department should organize the camps for free medical check-ups at the local level. This will help in early detection of the health related problem and its timely treatment as well as assessing further improvement or deterioration in health among the people suffering from the lifestyle related diseases.

*Availability of Free Medicines*

As the person suffering from these chronic conditions have to take treatment for rest of the life, so it becomes difficult for an ordinary person to manage these expenses. So, government should provide the free medicines for the needy people at primary health centers and government hospitals.

*Lifestyle Management*

Above all a healthy lifestyle is the most important way to prevent, curb and to cope up with the lifestyle related diseases. Healthy lifestyle includes the healthy diet, physical activity on regular basis, non-consumption of tobacco and tobacco products, avoidance of excessive use of alcohol etc.

Further, our study shows that doctors are not following preventive health guidelines to keep themselves healthy. So, in the present study, some suggestions are made for the medical fraternity in particular while keeping in mind the implications for them on the basis of findings of the present study.

**Suggestions for Medical Fraternity**

As we know, doctors are well learned strata of the society and completely aware about the causes, risk factors, preventive measures and coping strategies to manage the lifestyle related diseases. The following corrections can be suggested for doctors:

*Lifestyle Management Among Doctors*

- As in case of general public lifestyle management by taking low carbohydrates and low sugar diet taken at regular intervals can help in reducing the occurrence as well as the effect of lifestyle related diseases.

- Indulge in regular exercising and yoga in daily routines. Leisure time activities should also be not of sedentary nature as observed in the study.

- Night shifts and long working hours create a lot of biological and psychological issues with doctors, it is though an essential part of doctor's lifestyle but steps need to be taken to make sure proper rotation of doctors is done and adequate time is given for rest and other activities.

- Doctors should get themselves medically checked on routine basis. In the present study, it is seen that they often prescribe regular medical check-ups to their clients but they themselves pay least heed to it. Regular check-ups will help in detecting diseases in early stage and therefore take recourse to check them in advance.

*Stress Management*

The biggest reason cited for lifestyle related diseases by the unhealthy respondents (97/ 130) was stress. Therefore coping with the stress becomes the most important aspect of tackling lifestyle related diseases. The following can be considered as an efficient mechanism to deal with stress:

- Kinship ties are observed to be good at reducing stress. Even in the study, the ones with extended kinship ties were relatively less diseased. So doctors should be involved more in familial activities and functions. Collectively, it is seen as a great stress reducer and elicit good mood.

- Institutional mechanisms should be promoted to reduce the stressful environment at workplaces. For this purpose, weekly or monthly extra-curricular activities like singing, painting competition or may be physical fitness programmes like aerobics can be organized. Moreover, doctors should be encouraged to participate in them on regular basis

- Yoga or alternative activities can also help in reducing stress. Even small things like using stairs rather than elevators in work places can help if done regularly.

- Special workshops on stress management can be taken regularly for doctors dealing with high stress environment. For instance, ICU departments or IPDs etc.

Along with the above given suggestions, the following submission is to make changes in the curriculum of medical education. Doctors should be socialized to have humanistic approach while treating patients rather than having a mechanical orientation. This will be helpful in addressing a medical problem in holistic manner that will benefit not only the medical fraternity but also for the general public at large.

*Introduction of Behavior Sciences in Medical Science*

Since lifestyle and socio-cultural factors play an important role in the development of lifestyle related diseases, so doctors should be trained in behavior sciences for the better understanding of the causes of the lifestyle related diseases and their holistic treatment.

Doctors comprise the backbone of healthcare services. During their medical training they are educated to deal with the patient in parts not as a whole. So, only pathological parts of the patients are focused for treatment. Medical students should be motivated to have a humanistic approach for the diseased person rather than only focusing upon the symptoms of the disease. In this way, doctors will help in discovering the risks like dietary deficiencies, inadequate exercise, smoking, excessive use of alcohol and many more dangerous behaviors unknowingly going on in patients' lives.

**CONCLUSION**

The prevalence of lifestyle related diseases is increasing among all the sections of society in India.  This is primarily due to the presence of risk factors such as unhealthy diet, tobacco and alcohol consumption and lack of sufficient physical activity. These factors have penetrated in Indian society due to increase in consumerist culture in India. The opening of Indian markets and society due to global forces has contributed towards change in lifestyle of ordinary citizens.

Doctors in society play a pivot role in maintaining a healthy society. They are considered as 'Guardian of Health' in society. While fulfilling this role, doctors are expected to be in optimum health themselves. However, the present study reveals that doctors are not immune to the diseased state.  Moreover, it is witnessed that some of the doctors take their health and lifestyle casually.  The prime reasons for the lifestyle related diseases as highlighted by respondents were stress and sensitive nature of the job.  Thus the study showed that like other common people, doctors were as vulnerable to the lifestyle diseases such as diabetes, COPD, blood pressure etc.

As far as the psychological and social aspects are concerned,  some of doctors felt that it difficult to cope with the lifestyle related disease. They showed emotions like distress, anxiety and many even remained disturbed and their social activities with family and friends also got affected.  There seems to be minimal economic impact on the respondents as most of them belonged to higher income group.

This research brings back the focus on structure-agency debate, where the sociologists proposed that the both the structure and agency are important in understanding any social phenomenon.   The research is best described by the health lifestyle theory which prescribes that  the lifestyle habits of people are shaped by their social class.  The people of different social classes may however, exercise different lifestyle choices.  The doctors who follow a proper lifestyle management pattern remain healthy whereas others who continue to follow unhealthy lifestyle and  have one or more risk factors suffer from the lifestyle related diseases.

The study also confirms that genetic reasons are not the only reasons for lifestyle related diseases, so the lifestyle must be managed and efficient coping mechanism must be developed with the fold of society. Hence, insights brought forward by this research, a start can be made to help the medical community in managing the lifestyle related diseases, which in turn will be conducive in ushering a healthy and stress free society.

# REFERENCES

Abegunde, D. & Stanciole, A. (2006). *An estimation of the economic impact of chronic non-communicable diseases in selected countries.* World Health Organization (Working Paper): Department of Chronic Diseases and Health Promotion.

Abidi, N.F. (1992). *Social and professional roles: Study of female physician in Delhi govt. hospitals* (unpublished Ph.D. thesis). Department of Sociology, Jawahar Lal Nehru University, New Delhi.

Achidambaranathan, C. (2011). *A study on social practices associated with diseases among people living in coastal and inland villages in Tirunelveli district of Tamilnadu* (unpublished Ph.D. thesis). Department of Sociology, Manonmaniam Sundaranar University, Tirunelveli, India.

Advani, Mohan. (1980). *Doctor patient relationship in Indian hospital.* Jaipur: Sarghi Prakasan.

Alkerwi, Ala'a., Crichton, Georgina E. , Hébert, James R. (2015). Consumption of ready-made meals and increased risk of obesity: Findings from the observation of cardiovascular risk factors in Luxembourg (ORISCAV-LUX) study. *British Journal of Nutrition, 113*(2), 270-77.

Asif, M., Jameel, A., Sahito, N., Hwang, J., Hussain, A., Manzoor, F. (2019). Can leadership enhance patient satisfaction? Assessing the role of administrative and medical quality. *International Journal of Environmental Research and Public Health, 16*(17), 3212.

Ayas, N.T., White, D.P., Manson, J.E., Stampfer, M.J., Speizer, F.E., Malhotra, A., Hu, F.B. (2003). A prospective study of sleep duration and coronary heart disease in women. *Archives of Internal Medicine. 163*(2), 205-209.

Babu P, Suresh. (2017). *Adaptation to diabetes - A sociological study of diabetic patients in Kerala* (unpublished Ph.D. thesis). Department of Sociology, St. Teresa's college, Mahatma Gandhi Univesity, Ernakulam, Kerala.

Benziman, G., Kannai, R., & Ahmad, A. (2012).The wounded healer as cultural archetype. *CLCWeb: Comparative Literature and Culture, 14*(1), 2-9.

Bhardwaj, S.M. (1975). Attitude toward different systems of medicine: A survey of four villages in the Punjab-India. *Social Science and Medicine, 9*(11-12), 603-612.

Blumer, H. (1969). *Symbolic interactionism: Perspective and method.* Englewood Cliffs, New Jersey: Prentice Hall.

Bourdieu, P. (1984). *Distinction: A social critique of the judgement of taste.* London: Routledge.

Burton, W.N., Pransky, G., Conti, D. J., Chen, C.-Y., Edington, D.W. (2004). The association of medical conditions and presenteeism. *Journal of Occupational and Environmental Medicine, 46*(6), S38-S45.

Bury, M. (1991). The sociology of chronic illness: A review of research and prospects. *Sociology of Health and Illness, 13*(4), 451-68.

Caplan, R. D., Cobb, S., French, J.R.P., Harrison, R.V., Pinneau, S.R. (1975). *Job demands and worker health: Main effects and occupational difference.* U.S. Department of Health, Education and Welfare, DHEW (NIOSH) Publication No. 75-160, 1-353.

Carstairs, G.M. (1955). Medicine and faith in rural Rajasthan. In Paul, B. D. (Ed.), *Health culture and community.* New York : Russel Sage Foundation.

Chandani, Ambica (1980). *The Medical profession: A sociological exploration.* Delhi: Jain sons.

Cockerham, Wiiliam C. (1986). *Medical Sociology* (3rd ed.). Englewood Cliffs, New Jersey (USA): Prentice-Hall.

Cockerham, William C. (2000a). The sociology of health behavior and health lifestyles (pp. 159-72). In Chloe Bird, Peter Conrad, and Allen Fremont (Eds.), *Handbook of medical sociology* (5th ed.), Upper Saddle River, New Jersey: Prentice-Hall.

Cockerham, William C. (1998). *Medical Sociology* (7th ed.). Upper Saddler River, New Jersey: Prentice- Hall.

Cockerham, William C., (2005). Health lifestyle theory and the convergence of agency and structure. *Journal of Health and Social Behavior, 46*(1), 51-67.

Cockerham, William C., Alfred, R u tten. & Thomas, Abel. (1997). Conceptualizing contemporary health lifestyles: Moving beyond Weber. *Sociological Quarterly, 38*(2), 321-42.

Cockerham, William C., Snead, M. Christine, and DeWaal, Derek F. (2002). Health lifestyles in Russia and the socialist heritage. *Journal of Health and Social Behavior 43*(1), 42-55.

Coleman, D., & Iso-Ahola, S. E. (1993). Leisure and health: The role of social support and self-determination. *Journal of Leisure Research, 25*(2), 111-128.

*Collins English Dictionary online (2014).* Retrieved from https://www.harpercollins.com.au/9780007522743/collins-english-dictionary-12th-edition/

Compas, Bruce E., Jaser, Sarah S., Dunn, Madeleine J., Rodriguez, Erin M. (2012). Coping with chronic illness in childhood and adolescence. *Annual Review of Clinical Psychology, 8,* 455-480.

Conrad, Peter, & Kristin Barker. (2010). The social construction of illness: Key insights and policy implications. *Journal of Health and Social Behaviour, 51(S),* S67-S79.

Cooper, C., Rout, U., & Faragher, B. (1989). Mental health, job satisfaction and job stress among general practitioners. *BioMed Journal, 298*(6670), 366-70.

Dahlgren, G., & Whitehead, M. (1991). *Policies and strategies to promote social equity in health.* Background document to WHO-Strategy paper for Europe. Stockholm, Sweden: Institute for Futures Studies.

DeBenedette, Valerie. (2011, Nov. 29). *Doctor-patient relationship influences patient engagement.* Centre for Advancing Health (CFAH): Health Behaviour News Service.

Down To Earth. (2015, Sept. 17). *Eat at your own risk.* Retrieved from https://www.downtoearth.org.in/coverage/health/eat-at-your-own-risk-37902

Dubos, R. (1959). *Mirage of health: Utopias, progress, and biological change.* New York: Harper & Row.

Durkheim , Emile . (1966). *Suicide: A study in sociology.* Glencoe, IL: Free Press.

Eda, N. (2014). Yoga has beneficial effects on patients with chronic diseases and improves immune functions. *Journal of Clinical  Research and  Bioethics, 05*(05). Retrieved from: https://www.omicsonline.org/open-access/yoga-has-beneficial-effects-on-patients-with-chronicdiseases-and-improves-immune-functions-2155-9627.1000197.php?aid=32688

Eibl-Eibesfeldt, Irenaus. (1989). *Human ethology.* New York: Aldine de Gruyter.

Elstad, J. (1998). The psycho-social perspective on social inequalities in health. *Sociology of Health and Illness, 20*(5), 598-618.

Everson-Rose, Susan A., & Lewis, Tené T. (2005) Psychosocial factors and cardiovascular diseases. *Annual Review of Public Health, 26*, 469-500.

Ferguson, Warren J., & Candib, Lucy M. (2002). Culture, language and the doctor-patient relationship. *Family Medicine, 34* (5), 353-61.

Firth-Cozens, J. (2001). Interventions to improve physician's wellbeing and patient care. *Social Science & Medicine, 52*(2), 223-225.

Fitzpatrick, Kevin. & LaGory, Mark. (2000). *Unhealthy places: The ecology of risk in the urban landscape.* New York: Routledge.

Garelick, Antony I. (2012). Doctors health: Stigma and the professional discomfort in seeking help. *The  Psychiatrist (online), 36,* 81-84.

Gautam, Mamta., MacDonald, Rhona. (2001). Helping physicians cope with their own chronic illnesses. *West Journal of Medicine, 175*(5), 336-338.

Gerhardt, U. (1989). *Ideas about illness.* Houndsmill: Macmillan.

Germov, John. (2009). *Imagining health problems as social issues* (4th edition). United Kingdom: Oxford University Press. Retrieved from http://ogma.nemcastle.edu.au:8080/vital/access/manager/Repository/uon:8564.

Goffman, Erving . (1963). *Stigma: Notes on the management of spoiled identity.* Englewood Cliffs, New Jersey : Prentice-Hall.

Goffman, Erving. (1959). *The presentation of self in everyday life.* New York: Anchor.

Goodnow, J. J. (1990). The socialization of cognition: What's involved? In J. W. Stigler, R. A. Shweder, & G. Herdt (Eds.), *Cultural psychology: Essays on comparative human development* (pp. 259-286). New York: Cambridge University Press.

Gottlieb, D.J., Punjabi, N.M., Newman, A.B., Resnick, H.E., Redline, S., Baldwin, C.M., Nieto, F.J. (2005). Association of sleep time with diabetes mellitus and impaired glucose tolerance. *Archives of Internal Medicine, 165*(8), 863-67.

Gottlieb, D.J., Redline, S., Nieto, F.J., Baldwin, C.M., Newman, A.B., Resnick, H.E., Punjabi, N.M. (2006). Association of usual sleep duration with hypertension: The sleep heart health study. *Sleep, 29*(8), 1009-1014.

Govender, I., Mutunzi, E., Okonta, H.I. (2012). Stress among medical doctors working in public hospitals of the Ngaka Modiri Molema district, N-W province, South Africa. *South African Journal of Psychology, 18*(2), 42-46.

Government of India. (1998). *Indian nutrition profile.* Department of Woman and Child Development: Ministry of Human Resource Development. New Delhi: GOI

Ha, Jennifer Fong., & Longnecker, Nancy. (2010). Doctor-patient communication: A review. The *Ochsner Journal, 10*(1), 38-43.

Harris, Katherine M . (2003). How do patients choose physicians? Evidence from a national survey of enrollees in employment-related health plans. *Health Services Research, 38*(2), 711-32.

Hasan, H.A. (1979). *Medical sociology of rural India.* Ajmer: Sachin Publications.

Hegde, Shailendra Kumar B. , Vijayakrishnan, G., Sasankh, Akshaya K. , Venkateswaran, Sanjana. , Parasuraman, Ganeshkumar. (2016) . Lifestyle-associated risk for cardiovascular diseases among doctors and nurses working in a medical college hospital in Tamil Nadu, India. *Journal of Family Medicine Primary Care, 5*(2), 281-285.

Hinote, <u>Brian P.</u> (2015). William C Cockerham: The contemporary sociology of health lifestyles(Chapter 30, pp. 471-487) · *The Palgrave Handbook of Social Theory in Health, Illness and Medicine*. Available at doi: 10.1057/9781137355621_30·

Huggard, Peter., & Dixon, Robyn. (2011). "Tired of caring": The impact caring on resident doctors. *Australasian Journal of Disaster and Trauma Studies, 3,* 105-11.

Human and Health Services. (2014). *The health consequences of smoking-50 years of progress: A report of the surgeon general.* Retrieved from http://www.surgeongeneral.gov/library/reports/50-years-of-progress/.

Jaisal, Nand Lal. (1982). *Disease, treatment and society; A sociological analysis* (unpublished Ph.D. thesis). Centre for the Study of Social Systems, School of Social Sciences, Jawaharlal Nehru University, New Delhi.

Jardim, T.V., Sousa, A.L.L., Povoa, T.I.R., Barroso, W.K.S., Chinem, B., Jardim, L., Bernardes, R. Coca, A., Jardim, PCBV. (2015). The natural history of cardiovascular risk factors in health professionals: 20-year follow-up. *BioMed Central Public Health, 15*(1), 3-6.

Jaye, Chrystal., & Wilson, Hamish. (2003). When general practitioners become patients. *Health: An Interdisciplinary Journal for the Social Study of Health, Illness and Medicine, 7*(2), 201-225.

Johnson, J., Stewart, W., Hall, E., Fredlund, P. & Theorell, T. (1996). Long term psychosocial work environment exposure and cardio-vascular mortality among Swedish. *American Journal of Public Health, 86*(3), 334-331.

Joshi, Neela (1979). *Cultural factors in health- Studies in sociology of medicine in an Indian town* (unpublished Ph.D. thesis). Department of Anthropology and Sociology. University of Saugar. Sagar, Madya Pardesh.

Jovicic, A.D. (2015). Healthy eating habits among the population of Serbia: Gender and age differences. *Journal of Health, Population and Nutrition, 33*(1),76-84.

Juntunen, Juhani., Asp, Sisko., Olkinuora, Martti., Aarimaa, Markku., Strid, Leo., Kauttu, Kyllikki. (1988). Doctors drinking habits and consumption of alcohol. *BioMed Journal, 297.*

Kasasbeh, E., Chi, D.S., Krishnaswamy, G. (2006). Inflammatory aspects of sleep apnea and their cardiovascular consequences. *South Medical Journal, 99*(1), 58-67.

Kay, Margaret P., Michell, Geoffrey K., Del, Christopher B. (2004). Doctors do not adequately look after their own physical health. *Medical Journal of Australia, 181*(7), 368-370.

Kay, Margret., Clavarino, Alexandera., Doust, Jenny .(2008). Doctors as patients: A systematic review of doctors' health access and the barriers they experience. *The British Journal of General Practice, 58*(552), 501-508.

Kim, H.L., Park, H.J., Sim, Y.H., Choi, E.Y., Shim, K.W., Lee, S.W., Lee, H.S., Chun, H. (2016). Cancer prevalence among physicians in Korea: A single center study. *Korean Journal of Family Medicine, 37*(2), 91-96.

Kirkwood T. (1963). In S. Ibrahim, A. Kalache (eds), *Mechanisms of ageing in epidemiology in old age* (p. 3). London: BMJ Publishing Group.

Kleiber, D., & Nimrod, G. (2009). 'I can't be very sad': Constraint and adaptation in the leisure of a 'learning in retirement' group. *Leisure Studies, 28*(1), 67-83.

Kohatsu, N.D., Tsai, R., Young, T., Vangilder, R., Burmeister, L.F., Stromquist, A.M., Merchant, J.A. (2006). Sleep duration and body mass index in a rural population. *Archives of Internal Medicine, 166*(16), 1701-5.

Koopmanschap, M., Burdorf, A., Lötters, F. (2013). Work absenteeism and productivity loss at work. In Patric Loisal & Johannes Anema (eds), *Hand book of work disability-Prevention and management,* (1st ed.), pp. 31-41. New York: Springer-Verlag.

Kumar, Nikhilesh. (1986). *A sociological study of the medical profession* (unpublished Ph.D. thesis). Department of Sociology, The North-Eastern Hill University, Shillong.

Laskari, S., Pourzitaki C., Panagopoulou, E., Sardeli, C., Chourdakis,M., Papazisis, G., Kouvelas, D. (2010). Self-prescribing: A common phenomenon especially among young Greek doctors. *Review of Clinical Pharmacology and Pharmacokinetics International Edition, 24,* 166-167.

Lee, J.K., Grace, K.A., Taylor, A.J. (2006). Effect of a pharmacy care program on medication adherence and persistence, blood pressure, and low-density lipoprotein cholesterol: A randomized controlled trial. *Journal of American Medical Association (JAMA)*, *296*(21), 2563-2571.

Lerner, D., Amick III, B.C., Lee, J.C., Rooney, T., Rogers, W.H., Chang, H., Berndt, E.R. (2003). Relationship of employee-reported work limitations to work productivity. *Medical Care, 41(5)*, 649-659.

Lewy, R. (1986). Alcoholism in house staff physician: An occupational hazard. *Journal of Occupational Medicine, 28*(2), 79-81.

Lin, S-Y., Lin, C-L., Hsu, W-H., Wang, I-K., Chang, C-C., Huang, C-C., Kao, C-H., Liu, S-H.,  Sung, F-C. (2013). A comparison of cancer incidence among physician specialists and the general population: A Taiwanese cohort study. *Journal of Occupational Health. 55*(3), 158-166.

Link, B., & Phelan, J. (1995). Social conditions as fundamental causes of disease. *Journal of Health and Social Behavior,* extra issue, 80-94.

Livneh, H. & Antonak, R.F. (2005). Psychosocial adaptation to chronic illness and disability. *Journal of Counseling & Development, 83*(1), 12-20.

Lobelo, F., Duperly, J., Frank, E. (2009). Physical activity habits of doctors and medical students influence their counseling practices. *British Journal of Sports Medicine, 43*(2), 89-92.

Lockley, Steven W., Barger, Laura K., Ayas, Najib T., Rothschild, Jeffrey M., Czeisler, Charles A., Landrigan, Christopher P. (2007). Effects of healthcare provider work hours and sleep deprivation on safety and performance. *The Joint Commission Journal on Quality and Patient Safety, 33*(11), 7-18.

Madan T.N. (1980). *Doctors and society.* New Delhi: Vikas Publishing House Pvt. Ltd.

Madan, T.N. (1972). Doctors in north Indian city: Recruitment, role perception and role performance in Satish Sabbarwal (ed.), *Beyond the village- Sociological exploration*. Simla: Indian Institute of Advanced Study.

Mahato, Raj Kishore., &  Suman, Parineeta. (2013). Good doctor-patient relationship: Its status in clinical practice. *Scholars Journal of Applied Medical Sciences, 1*(4), 359-362.

Malathi, A., Damodaran, A. (1999). Stress due to exams in medical students- Role of yoga. *Indian Journal of Physiology and Pharmacology, 43*(2), 218-224.

Malathi, M.S. (1993). *Medical Sociology: Social epidemiology and illness behaviour- A study of cancer cervix* (unpublished Ph.D. thesis). Department of Sociology, Shri Krishnadevaraya University, Anantapur.

Marriot, McKim. (1955). *Western medicine in a village of northern India*. New York: Russell Sage Foundation.

Maruyama, S., Kohno, K., & Morimoto, K. (1995). A study of preventive medicine in relation to mental health among middle-management employees (Part 2). *Japanese Journal of Hygiene, 50*(4), 849-860.

Mathur, Indu. (1975). *Interrelation in an organisation*. Jaipur: Alekh Publishers.

McAmmond, D. (2000). *Food and nutrition surveillance in Canada: An environmental scan*. Ottawa, ON: Health Canada.

McKall, K. (2001). An insider's guide to depression. *BioMedical Journal, 323*(7319), 1011.

McKeown, T. (1979). *The role of medicine: Dream, mirage or nemesis* (2nd ed.). Oxford: Basil Blackwell.

Mckevitt, C. & Morgan, M. (1997). Illness does not belong to us. *Journal of Royal Society of Medicine, 90*(9), 491-95.

McQuaide, M. (2005).The rise of alternate health care: A sociological account. *Social Theory, 3*(4), 286-301.

Mead , George H. (1934) . *Mind, self, and society*. Chicago : University of Chicago Press .

Menon, Anitha., & Munalula, Betyy. (2007). Stress in doctors: A pilot study of the university teaching hospital, Lusaka, Zambia. *Journal of Psychology in Africa. 17*(1), 137-140.

Minocha, Anita. (1974). *Some aspect of the social system of an Indian hospital* (unpublished Ph.D. thesis), Delhi University, Delhi.

Minocha, Anita. (1996). *Perceptions and interactions in a medical setting: A sociological study of women's hospital.* New Delhi: Hindustan Publishing Corporation.

Mishra, Chander Kant .(1994). *Doctors and their professional world view: A study of ayurvedic and allopathic doctors in the city of Varanasi* (unpublished Ph.D. thesis). Jawaharlal Nehru University, New Delhi: India.

Montgomary, A..J. (2011). A review of self-medication in physician and medical students. *Occupational Medicine, 61*(7), 490-497.

Mukund, Malini (2002). *A sociological study of heart diseases* (unpublished Ph.D. thesis). Department of Sociology. Manglore university.

Murray, J., Craig C.L., Honey, S., House, A. (2012). A systematic review of patient reported factors associated with uptake and completion of cardiovascular lifestyle behaviour change. *BMC Cardiovascular Disorders, 12*, 120.

Nagla, Madhu. (1990). *A Sociological study of medical profession: A study of medical organisation and profession of medicine in Haryana* (unpublished Ph.D. thesis). Department of Sociology, Jawaharlal Nehru University, New Delhi: India.

Najman, J. (1980). Theories of disease causation and the concept of general susceptibility: A review. *Social Science & Medicine, 14*(3), 231-37.

National Commission on Macroeconomics and Health. (1996-2016). *Report on COPD.* Ministry of Health and Family Welfare, New Delhi.

National Heart, Lung and Blood Institute . (2011). *Your guide to sleep habit.* U.S. Department of Health and Human Services: National Institutes of Health.

National Institute of Diabetes, Digestive and Kidney Diseases. (NIDDK, 2015). *Health risks of being overweight.* U.S. Department of Health and Human Services: National Institutes of Health. Available at   https://www.niddk. nih.gov/about-niddk

National Programme for Prevention and Control of Cancer, Diabetes. Cardiovascular diseases and Stroke (NPCDCS). (2007). Ministry of Health and Family Welfare, Government of India.

National Restaurant Association. (2012). *Facts at a glance.* Retrieved from http://www.restaurant.org/research/facts.

National Sample Survey Organisation. (NSSO, 2006). *Morbidity, health care and the conditions of aged* (Report No.507). Ministry of Statics and Programme Implementation, GOI.

Newman, S., Steed, L. & Mulligan, K. (2004). Self-management interventions for chronic illness. *Lancet, 364,* 1523-1537.

Nikolic, Irina A.,  Stanciole, Anderson E. & Zaydman, Mikhail.(2011). *Chronic emergency: Why NCDs matter.* World Bank Health, Nutrition and Population Discussion Paper.

Nilsson, P.M., Nilson, J.A., Ostergren, P.O., Berglund, G. (2005). Social mobility, marital status, and mortality risk in an adult life course perspective: The Malmo Preventive Project. *Scandinavian   Journal of Public Health, 33*(6), 412-23.

Oommen, T.K. (1978). *Doctors and nurses : A study in occupational role structure.* Delhi: Mcmillan.

Parsons, T. (1951) The social system. London: Routledge.

Parsons, T. (1978). *Action theory and the human condition.* New York: Free Press.

Philibert, Ingrid. (2005). Sleep loss and performance in residents and non-physicians: A meta-analytic examination. *Sleep, 28*(11), 1392-1402.

Polonsky, W.H.,  Anderson, Barbara J., Lohrer, Patricia A., Welch, Garry., Jacobson, Alan M., Aponte, Jennifer E., Schwartz, Carolyn E. (1995). Assessment of diabetes-related distress. *Diabetes Care, 18(6)*, 754-760.

Popkin, B. M. (2002). The shift in stages of the nutritional transition in the developing world differs from past experiences! *Public Health Nutrition, 5*(1A), 205-214.

Post Graduate Institute of Medical Education and Research. (PGIMER, 2014). *Burden of NCD risk factors in Punjab State*. Department of Community Medicine, Chandigarh.

Prabakar, S. (2010). *Problems of people living with chronic disease – A sociological analysis* (unpublished Ph.D. thesis). Department of Sociology, School of Social Sciences and International Studies. Pondicherry University, Puducherry.

Pressman, S., Matthews, K. A., Cohen, S., Martire, L. M., Scheier, M., Baum, A., & Schulz, R. (2009). Association of enjoyable leisure activities with psychological and physical well-being. *Psychosomatic Medicine, 71*(7), 725-732.

Price, R.A., Elliott, M.N., Zaslavsky, A.M., Hays, R.D., Lehrman, W.G., Rybowski, L.,.....Cleary, P. D. (2014) Examining the role of patient experience surveys in measuring health care quality. *Medical   Care Research and  Review, 71*(5), 522-54.

Purohit, M., Verma, K. (2016).  Prevalence of non-communicable diseases in doctors. *International Journal of Innovative Research and Review, 4(2), 54-61.*

Rammanna, A. & Bambawale, Usha. (1978). Occupational attitude of patients. *Sociological Bulletin, 2*(2), 190-207.

Ray, Kausik (2011). *Level of awareness and access to the treatment of cancer : A sociological study among the patients in West Bengal* (unpublished Ph.D. thesis). Department of Sociology, University of North Bengal, Raja Ram mohanpur district, Darjeeling.

Rayomand, Engineer. (2018, August 9). How much milk is too much: A nutritionist debunks myths we all have! *The Better India*. Retrieved from https://www.thebetterindia.com/155455/milk-benefits-nutritionist-news/

Robles, Theodore F., & Kiecolt-Glaser, Janice K. (2003). The Physiology of marriage: Pathways to health. *Physiology and Behavior, 79*(3), 409-16.

Royer, A. (1998). *Social isolation: The most distressing consequence of chronic illness*. Retrieved from http://research.allacademic.com/meta/p_mla_apa_research_citation/1/1/0/2/1/p110216_index.html?phpsessid=7fc502fc26e39b3c7a03341b5cc8d2b1.

Ruhm, C. (2000). Are recessions good for your health? *Quarterly Journal of Economics, 115*(2), 616-650.

Schlicht, S. M., Gordon, I.R., Ball, J.R., Christie, D.G. (1990). Suicide and related deaths in Victorian doctors. *Medical Journal of Australia, 153*(9), 518-521.

Schmidt, Harald. (2016, April 13). Chronic disease prevention and health promotion (Chapter 5). In D.H. Barrett, L. W. Ortmann, A. Dawson et al. (Eds.), *Public health ethics: Cases spanning the globe (online),*. Cham (CH): Springer. Retrieved from https://www.ncbi.nlm.nih.gov/books/NBK435779/

Schulz, S., Einsle, F., Schneider, N., Wensing, M., & Gensichen,, J. (2016). Illness behavior of general practitioners- A cross-sectional study. *Occupational Medicine (London), 67*(1), 33-37.

Shabbir, A., Malik, S.A., Malik, S.A. (2016). Measuring patients' healthcare service quality perceptions, satisfaction, and loyalty in public and private sector hospitals in Pakistan. *International Journal of Quality and Reliability Management, 33(5)*, 538-557.

Singh, Sawarn. (2013). *Economics of morbidity in Punjab: Causes and consequences.* India: Dorling Kindersley Pvt. Ltd.

Sox, H.C. (2013, June 19). The health checkup: Was it ever effective? Could it be effective? *Journal of American Medical Association (JAMA), 309*(23), 2496-7.

Srivastava, A.L. (1979). *Human relations in social organisation*. Allahabad: Chugh.

St-Onge, M.P., Ard, J., Baskin, M.L., Chiuve, S.E., Johnson, H.M., Kris-Etherton, P., Varady K .(2017). Meal timing and frequency: Implications for cardiovascular disease prevention. A scientific statement from the American Heart Association (Circulation). *PubMed, 135*(9), e96-e121.

Straus, R. (1957) The nature and status of medical sociology. *American Sociological Review, 22* (2), 200-4.

The World Health Report *(1998). Life in the 21st century: A vision for all.* Geneva: WHO.

Thompson, W. T, Cupples, M., Sibbert, C.H., Skan, D.I., Bradley, T. (2001). Challenge of culture, conscience and contract to general practitioner's care of their own health: Qualitative study. *BioMedical Journal, 323*(7315),728-731.

Tiwari, Ruby. (1999). *Socio-cultural dimensions of doctor-patient interactions under different medical systems in the metropolitan setting of Delhi* (unpublished Ph.D. thesis). Centre for the study of social systems, School of Social Sciences, Jawaharlal Nehru University, New Delhi.

Tomlinson, Jonantham. (2014, June 02). Lessons from "the other side": Teaching and learning from doctor's illness narratives. *BMJ, 348.* Retrieved from doi: https://doi.org/10.1136/bmj.g3600

Turner, Jane., Kelly, Brian. (2000). Emotional dimensions of chronic disease. *Western Journal of Medicine, 172*(2), 124-128.

Tuthill, J.L., Ahmed, M.S., Mathewe, G., Balton, A.C., Molokhia, A.A. (2013). Work-related stress amongst doctors in intensive care, anesthetics, accident and emergency and general medicine. *BioMed Central, 17*(2).

U.S. Department of Health and Human Services. (2018). *Physical activity guidelines for Americans.* A scientific report by HHS: Office of Disease Prevention and Health Promotion.

Umberson, Deborah. (1987). Family status and health behaviors: Social control as a dimension of social integration. *Journal of Health and Social Behavior, 28*(3), 306-319.

Umberson, Debra. & Montez, Jennifer Karas. (2010). Social relationships and health: A flashpoint for health policy. *Journal of Health and Social Behaviour, 51,* S54-S66.

Umberson, Debra. (1992). Gender, marital status and the social control of health behaviour. *Social Science and Medicine, 34* (8), 907-17.

Vachon, M.L.S. (1995). Staff stress in hospice/palliative care: A review. *Palliative Medicine, 9*(2), 91-122.

Varì, Rosaria., Scazzocchio, Beatrice. , D'Amore, Antonio., Giovannini, Claudio. , Gessani, Sandra., Masella, Roberta. (2016). Gender-related differences in lifestyle may affect health status. *Ann Ist Super Sanità Journal, 52*(2), 158-166.

Veblen, Thorstein. (1899). *The theory of the leisure class: An economic study of institutions.* New York: Random House.

Velankanni, I. (2014). *A sociological study on systems of medicine and its use in urban setting in Madurai district* (unpublished Ph.D. thesis). Department of Sociology, Madurai Kamaraj University, Madurai.

Venkatratnam, R. (1979). *Medical sociology in an Indian setting.* Madras: Macmillan.

Volpato, S., Blaum, C., Resnick, H., Ferrucci, L., Fried, L.P., Guralnik, J.M. & Women's Health and Aging Study. (2002). Co-morbidities and impairments explaining the association between diabetes and lower extremity disability: The women's health and aging study. *Diabetes Care, 25*(4), 678-683.

Wada, Koji., Yoshikawa, Toru., Goto, Takahisa., Hirai, Aizan., Matsushima, Eisuke., Nakashima, Yoshifumi., Akaho, Rie., Kido, Michiko., Hosaka, Takashi. (2011). Lifestyle habits among physicians working at hospitals in Japan. *Japan Medical Association Journal, 54*(5), 318-324.

Walker, A. E. (2007). Multiple chronic diseases and quality of life: Patterns emerging from a large national sample, Australia. *Chronic Illness, 3*(3), 202-218.

Warburton, D.E., Nicol, C.W., Bredin, S.S. (2006). Health benefits of physical activity: The evidence. *Canadian Medical Association Journal, 174*(6), 801-9.

Weber, M. (1921). *Wirtschafft und Gesselchaft*. Tubingen: Mohr.

Weber, Max. (1978). *Economy and society*. Guenther Roth and Claus Wittich (eds.) (1st ed.), pp. 956-1005. New York: Bedminister Press.

Weiss, Mitchell G., Ramakrishna, Jayashree., & Somma, Daryl. (2006). Health-related stigma: Rethinking concepts and interventions. *Psychology, Health & Medicine, 11*(3), 277-287.

Wessely, Alex. & Gerada, Clare. (2013).*When doctors need treatment : An Anthropological approach to why doctors make bad patients.* Retrieved from http://careers.bmj.com/careers/advice/view-article.html?id=20015402

White, Kevin. (2002). *An introduction to the sociology of health and illness.* London: Sage Publications.

Whittemore, Robin & Dixon, Jane (2008). Chronic illness: The process of integration. *Journal of Clinical Nursing, 17*(0), 177-187. doi: 10.1111/j.1365-2702.2007.02244.x

Willett, Walter C., Koplan, Jeffrey P., Nugent, Rachel., Dusenbury, Courtenay., Puska, Pekka., & Gaziano, Thomas A. (2006). Prevention of chronic disease by means of diet and lifestyle changes (Chapter 44). In D.T. Jamison, J.G. Breman, A.R. Measham, et al. (Eds.), *Disease Control Priorities in Developing Countries* (2nd edition). New York: Oxford University Press. Retrieved from https://www.ncbi.nlm.nih.gov/books/NBK11795/#__NBK11795_dtls__

Wiskar, Katie. (2012). Physician health: A review of life style behavior and preventive health care among physicians. *British Columbia Medical Journal, 54*(8), 419-423.

Wond, Josephine GWS. (2008, June). Doctors and stress. *Medical Bulletin, 13*(6).

Wong, Samuel Y.S., & Lee, Albert. (2006). Communication skill and doctor-patient relationship. *Medical Bulletin, II* (3).

World Health Organization (WHO, 2002). *Diet, physical activity and health.* Geneva : WHO.

World Health Organization. (WHO, 1946). *Constitution of World Health Organization*. Geneva: WHO

World Health Organization. (WHO, 1999). *Global status report on alcohol*. Geneva: WHO

World Health Organization. (WHO, 1999). *Global strategy for prevention of and control of non-communicable diseases*. Geneva: WHO.

World Health Organization. (WHO, 2002). *Reducing risks, promoting healthy life*. Geneva: WHO.

World Health Organization. (WHO, 2002).*Globalization, diets, and NCDs*. Geneva: WHO.

World Health Organization. (WHO, 2003). *Diet, nutrition, and the prevention of chronic diseases*. Report of a joint WHO/FAO expert consultation. Geneva (WHO Technical Report Series, No. 916).

World Health Organization. (WHO, 2005). *WHO STEPS surveillance manual: The WHO STEP-wise approach to chronic disease risk factors surveillance*. Geneva: WHO.

World Health Organization. (WHO, 2005a). *Preventing chronic diseases: A vital investment*. WHO Global Report. Geneva: WHO.

World Health Organization. (WHO, 2010). *Global recommendations on physical activity for health*. Geneva: WHO.

World Health Organization. (WHO, 2011). *The world conference on social determinants of health, Brazil*. Geneva: World Health Organization. Available at http://www.who.int/sdhconference/declaration/en/ i-morbidity and equity in the WHO Eastern Mediterranean Region.

World Health Organization. (WHO, 2011a). *Global status report on non-communicable diseases 2010*. Geneva: WHO.

World Health Organization. (WHO, 2014). *Burden of NCDs and their risk factors in India: Excerpted from global status report on non-communicable diseases*. Geneva: WHO.

Xavier, D., Pais, P., Devereaux, P. J., Xie, C., Prabhakaran, D., Reddy, K. S. (2008). Treatment and outcomes of acute coronary syndromes in India (CREATE): A prospective analysis of registry data. *Lancet, 371*(9622), 1435-42.

Yaccob, Ismail., Abdullah, Zainal Abidin. (1993). Smoking habits and attitudes among doctors in a Malaysian hospital. *South Asian Journal Tropical Medicine Public Health. 24*(1), 28-31.

Young, P.V. (1956). *Scientific social survey and research.* New York: Asia Publishing House.

Ziglio, E., Currie, C., & Rasmussen, V.B. (2004). The WHO cross-national study of health behavior in school aged children from 35 countries: Findings from 2001–2002. *Journal of School Health, 74*(6), 204-206.